MW00937526

When life hands you pink lemons:

Making the best out of early stage breast cancer

Nicole Briamonte-Malato

Copyright © 2012 Nicole E. Malato
All rights reserved.
ISBN-13: 978-1480035997

ISBN-10: 1480035998

DEDICATION

This book is dedicated to:

- My husband who is the partner in life I could ask for. Thank you for loving me through this nonsense. You are one of a kind. Love you more than words can say.

- My son: on the day I was diagnosed, I wondered why God would let a mother with a 2 year old face this challenge. On the day after my diagnosis, I realized why. Your smile, joyful spirit and resilience are my fuel to keep fighting.

- My mom who started this journey as my biggest supporter, and then ended up taking her own journey as well. You made me proud as you fought with grace.

- My dad for always being a man of faith and courage, even when watching his two best girls battle cancer.

- My brothers: Frank for being my cheerleader, always encouraging my writing and pretty much everything else, Chris for always knowing just what to say and when to say it. You don't say much, but when you pick your spots, they are always perfect, and Rick for being my comic relief and friend always.

- My ladies for being the best friends a girl ask for, thank you for loving me unconditionally, just the way I am.

- Courtney and Nancy, my two personal nurse case managers. I appreciate your willingness to discuss topics no family member should ever have to talk about! Your support and knowledge made my journey so much easier.

- The rest of team Angels. I was blessed with the most amazing cheering squad. Every one of you helped in some way. I love you!

- And finally, God, I will continue to keep the faith, and make the best of any challenges that come my way.

CONTENTS

ACKNOWLEDGMENTS

I want to thank all of the wonderful people out there who have changed the face of cancer, those who have made strides in treatment and in survivorship. I am eternally grateful for those who have dedicated their lives to research and science, always in search of the cure. I also want to acknowledge the Cancer Support Community in Eatontown, especially SVF, for being the part of my treatment that healed my soul. You made this journey a beautiful one by showing me that life with cancer is still joyous and vibrant!

FOREWORD

When my kid sister was first diagnosed with breast cancer at the age of 34, it quite literally knocked the wind out of me. I was returning from a business trip when I got the news, and I remember feeling numb and short of breath as I walked through Chicago's O'Hare International Airport – just hoping I wouldn't break down in front of a bunch of strangers.

The next few weeks were a whirlwind of emotions for the entire family. Everyone tried to do all they could to be strong for Nicole and provide support and strength. But as things progressed, a funny thing happened – it became clear that she was helping all of us far more than we were helping her.

I write for a living and so just before her surgery, I dealt with my emotions the best way I knew how – by putting pen to paper to detail all the reasons why I knew my little sister would win her battle with cancer. Here's what I wrote …

Why We Know She Will Beat You

- You, cancer, are weakness; my sister is strength.

- You are deceitful; she is open and honest.
- You hide from sight; she faces things head on.
- You are ugly; she is graceful.
- You work alone; she has a posse (a really big, loud, formidable posse).
- You prey on fear; she is courage.
- You tear things down; she builds them up.
- You are darkness; she is light.
- You are vile; she is kind.
- You are despair; she has faith
- You are despised; she is loved.

A year and a half later, my sister has turned her battle with cancer into beacon of light for so many others. Through her blog and other writings she has inspired cancer survivors around the world to have faith and be strong. In the pages of this book, you will find all the strength, grace and courage my sister has displayed every day in this fight. All invaluable assets when facing any challenge life can throw at you.

I am proud to be Nicole Malato's brother. As you read these pages, you will understand why.

-- Frank Briamonte III

1. MAKING PINK LEMONADE

You know what they say: when life hands you lemons, you should make lemonade.

But what if you just don't like lemonade?

It may fluster you at first, but you can still find good use for those lemons. You can always make lemon meringue pie, lemon ice, lemon chicken, lemon drop shots, or citrus margaritas. I have even heard that lemon juice can help remove lime scale around faucets. Who knew? Or if none of these work for you, you just can take the lemon and throw it at a person who is ticking you off.

Truth be told, everyone encounters some adversity or proverbial lemons in their lives. Admittedly, some folks seem to get as larger share than others, but each person gets it to a varying degree. However, there is no denying that every person will find themselves at the foot of some mountain that seems too high to climb at some point in their life. It's what we do with those challenges that makes all of the difference. At the end of the day, we all have many choices to make. Some of those may be more tangible decisions in terms of what path we will take, whether that be medical treatment options, career changes, or confronting a bully. Some of those choices, however, are more introspective in nature, and about how we will allow those challenges to affect our lives, and what sort of outcome we will get from it.

The point is, when a lemon comes your way, don't let it wither on your counter to become nothing more than fodder for fruit flies. Do something with it! We all have the ability to take something bitter and make it something sweet. Sometimes, it may seem impossible at first, but persistence only makes the end result even sweeter.

I guess you could say I was fortunate. My biggest lemon in life waited until I was 34 to come flying at me, smacking me in the side of the head out of nowhere. I was blindsided. I can only assume that perhaps because it waited that long to appear in my life, it had to be a doozy: I was diagnosed with stage 2b breast cancer. Not only was it a huge lemon, it was pink! What can a girl do with that?

I was stunned. I had no history of breast cancer in my family. I have a really staggering statistic for you. Pay attention because it's an important one: 85% of the women who are diagnosed with breast cancer have no family history[i]. I am one of those 85%. Think about this on the flip side: only 15% of women diagnosed have a family history. Yes, really! So when you think to yourself, "I don't have to worry. I am not at risk for breast cancer because it's not in my family", I'm sorry to be the one to tell you, but you may just be wrong. I thought that for many years. Right up until May 3rd, 2011.

Nothing in this world makes you consider your own mortality (especially in your mid-30s) like a cancer diagnosis. However, there is a gift in that realization. Sometimes, it's hard to recognize, so I will tip you off on what it is. While most people take their lives and health for granted (including me prior to May 2011), someone diagnosed with cancer does not. We are given the unique opportunity to really explore what sort of impact we would like to make in this world. So, ask yourself, what legacy do you want to leave? Then spend your time on this earth making your mark on this world. Let the world be a better place because you are in it regardless of the trauma you encounter. Find your own recipe to make lemonade. For me, this book is my big, cool, refreshing pitcher.

When I realized that the vast majority of women who get this diagnosis have no family history, and many of them were gliding through life, as I was, thinking they have no risk, I decided to make it my mission to spread the word. To say that I hate that I was diagnosed with cancer is an understatement, but there was nothing I can do to change that fact. However, I could either sit here and pretend like it didn't happen to me, and that I can't make a difference in this world, or I could do something about it, and change it into a positive outcome. I decided to pour a little lemonade out into the world. I can educate people, make other women's journey through breast cancer a little easier by sharing my experiences and tips I learned along my way. Perhaps I can even save someone's life by educating others. That would be a miracle in and of itself. It is possibilities like that which make my home-brewed pink lemonade naturally sweet!

Please note that I am not a doctor by any stretch of the imagination so I will not give medical advice. I am nowhere near qualified enough for that. My intention is to share with you what it is like to look at life through the eyes of a survivor. I have learned a lot in the months following my diagnosis, and I want to share that knowledge. As such, I tell my story, hopefully invoke a couple of laughs, and provide you with some suggestions for coping and managing this beastly experience, both physically and emotionally. As I navigated my way through the complicated world of breast cancer, I relied heavily on the advice of other survivors. They gave me much comfort by validating my experience and giving me ideas that I hadn't thought of to help manage the side effects. It is my hope to pay that kindness forward through this book.

The book is structured such that the chapters are predominantly focused on the various phases of the breast cancer journey. This was done intentionally because I know that breast cancer can be such an overpowering experience. Women who are going through treatment can focus on each component as it comes rather than overwhelm themselves. As I was working on the book, several wonderful women I knew went through this as well. As they hit each various stage, I shared with them the applicable chapter to help give them a sense of what to expect. However you choose to read this is fine with me. My prayer is that it helps you in your journey.

So sit back and drink up!

2. SURVIVING THE DIAGNOSIS

Nothing can prepare you for it. It's one of those life-changing moments where someone flips a switch and suddenly the world is upside-down and inside-out all at once. You usually don't see it coming. Even though I had gone for the biopsy 24 hours earlier, I wasn't ready. I suppose no one ever is. I just never believed it would happen to me.

Prior to May 2011, I was the least scientific person you could ever meet. I somehow managed to get through high school, college and graduate school without taking a single day of Anatomy/Physiology. I had avoided the typical coming of age ritual of dissecting anything in Biology. Looking back, to this day, I am not sure how I got out of it, but being a queasy person, I guess I am not surprised. Perhaps it was self-preservation. No one wants to be that girl who passes out over a sliced open frog corpse. Suffice it to say, when it comes to knowledge of my own body, I was self-taught, and knew very little about anything medically-related.

Up until my diagnosis, I was in good health. I had no chronic health issues. My biggest medical challenge was keeping my seasonal allergies under control. I have never smoked a single cigarette in my life, and consumed alcohol very limitedly. I exercised 3 times a week. I tried to ensure that I ate sufficient fruits and veggies. I took a multivitamin on a fairly regular basis. I was diligent about going to annual well-patient visits. As far as anyone could tell, I had a very low risk of getting this disease. Out of curiosity, following the diagnosis, I did several online breast health risk calculators. I wanted to see if I was missing something glaring in my lifestyle that would have put me at risk. They all showed me as having between 5 and 15% risk of getting breast cancer in my lifetime, never mind as a young adult. I am thankful that when I felt a lump in my right breast, I knew that the wise thing to do would be to talk to my doctor.

If you have not been diagnosed with breast cancer and are just reading the book for your own information, learn from me the importance of being proactive. I want people to know what to look for in case you should find something unusual. Self-exams are so very important, especially if you are under the age of 40 as there is very little screening available to you. There are plenty of resources available in print and online regarding how to do self-exams. Read them and learn your body. It's your best defense.

I have to admit, I found the first lump by accident (it turns out I had 1 in the right breast and 4 in the left. Yikes!). I was laying on the floor with my son, and reached over to scratch an itch on the side of my boob and there it was! The lump in the right side was clearly a lump. The best description I can give is to say that it felt like a very small pebble was under the skin stuck in the breast tissue. Depending on the size, a tumor could feel like a grain of rice, a stone, a pea, a bean, or even something larger. The left side, which ended up actually being a slightly higher stage than the right did not quite have the same palpable lump that was one the other side. There were a few sections where the tissue felt thicker, denser, but it wasnothing that I would have been alarmed about had it been the only thing I felt. As it turns out, there were several small diffused clusters of cancer on that side, which made them harder to detect.

I was not as diligent about doing self-exams as I could have been because I foolishly figured I was low-risk. I wish I had been more concerned because perhaps I would have found it in an earlier stage and managed to avoid the trauma of chemotherapy. I have no idea how long this invader was hanging out in my body, nor how long the tumor was palpable. There is nothing I can do to change that fact in my life. However, you can learn from this, do your self-exams regularly and know what is normal for your body. Do not hesitate to talk to you doctor at any time if you have questions or have concerns. I cannot stress this enough: if you find something, bring it up to your doctor. You are not being paranoid, you are being smart!

Upon finding the lump, I called my doctor pretty quickly. Here is what I expected to happen: I would go to my Gynecologist (which I did). She would tell me that she was sending me in to have it looked at, but would assure me not to worry, that it was likely nothing to be concerned about (which she did). I would take the afternoon off of work, go for my mammogram, and go treat myself to a little retail therapy when I was done (two out of three of which happened). I expected that they would tell me I would have to routinely go back for mammograms, assuming there would be something benign there that they would want to watch (this did not happen). I was so sure that this would be a no brainer, that I told my husband not to come with me and insisted I would be fine.

So I arrived, expecting this to be a normal quick visit, but it snow-balled rather quickly. After my second mammogram that day, they sent me immediately into a follow-up ultrasound. Seeing the look on my technician's face told me what I did not see coming. The best way to describe her expression was the "oh shit" face. She wasn't allowed to tell me what she saw because she was not a doctor herself, but her nonverbal cues said it all. Something was very wrong. It is never a good sign when they are doing a diagnostic ultrasound and they click a lot or they wear the "oh shit" face! They sent me immediately into biopsy. At the time, I was upset that they rushed it, but in my heart, I knew I was only upset because it was clear they were rushing because it was not good news.

The biopsy was of course painful. That was exacerbated by the fact that I was crying and terrified. I was hoping they would knock me out because I wasn't sure if I could handle it, but no dice. I was awake for the whole thing. I watched the screen as they repeatedly stuck me with a long needle and went in to excavate tissue samples. It kind of looked like pac-man on the screen, I thought to myself, slightly amused. You could see on the screen the little device inching closer to the tumor, and then eventually munching away at the black hole on the screen. I might have found this to be more fun if it pac-man wasn't chomping on cancer.

Admittedly, I was pleased by how the breast center handled my case. It was nice to be treated as high priority, but admittedly, it unnerved me because I didn't want to be the one who required such attention. Before all the chaos started, I thought it was nice that they give every woman a pink rose for their appointment. As the day wore on, I joked that the whole experience was like a bad date. They give you a flower, and then awkwardly squish your boobs. Of course, by the end of my hectic day, I informed them that they should have given me a dozen roses and a bottle of wine, or treat me to dinner after everything they put me through. Truth be told, they handled me with the utmost kindness and professionalism. As scary as it was, I found myself surrounded by caring women. Their concern was evident, and that did provide me some comfort through a very harrowing afternoon. It would have been nice if the concern was unwarranted.

Unfortunately, within 24 hours, I got that call. My life changed forever.

Shock doesn't cover the emotion that I felt when I heard my radiologist say over the phone "You have cancer". Terror, sadness, disbelief, anger, worry, even guilt flooded through me in those first moments. The best way to describe the physical sensation that occurs when you hear those words is to say that it felt like someone took a giant bucket of ice water and poured it down my insides. The worst part was that it seemed like the ice took a long time to melt in there. I certainly didn't ask for this in my life, but here I was, suddenly counted among the 2.5 million women living with breast cancer in the United States. I was part of a club of beautiful, vibrant women, a club that I greatly admired and respected, but one I did not want to be a part of myself.

To be honest, I couldn't recount to you with great accuracy what happened in the hours and days following the news. I remember my husband walking in moments after I got the news. I am not sure I even told him what the doctor said: I didn't have to. We just cried and held onto each other right there in the kitchen. Slowly, I informed the people closest to me. I know that my family arrived promptly, and there were a lot of red, puffy eyes. I know that my phone rang incessantly as word made its way through my social network. The night I got diagnosed, I felt like I couldn't remember how to sleep, and was afraid that I wouldn't know how to go through my daily routine the next day. This was the very first time when I realized (and admittedly struggled with) knowledge that I was going to need a lot of support to manage all that was coming my way.

You will see this as a recurring theme throughout the book: let people help you. If you are like me, you are used to taking care of everyone else. This shift is a huge challenge to accept, but it will make things more manageable if you learn to reach out and ask for help. There are some things people can do right away to assist you. When you get your diagnosis, calling everyone who you want to know your situation can be a very overwhelming task. It's unrealistic to think you can do that on your own. So it's ok to appoint people to set up a phone chain and spread the news for you. You may not be ready to speak to everyone at this point, and that is perfectly ok. I do feel that the more people that know, the more people can support you, and the support will help boost your spirits when you need it most. However, don't feel like you need to add the role of broadcaster to your job description, let someone else handle that. Give someone a list, and let them have at it. It will be one less taxing chore for you, and they will feel relieved to be able to help you in some way.

I have often likened the early days in the new cancer life as living in a snow globe. It felt to me like I was standing in the middle of this tiny, serene world, and some child picked up my little world and shook it violently. I stood there, frozen, watching all these little white pieces of crap just flying around chaotically, stunned by what had happened to my previously blissfully benign existence. It was confusing, overwhelming and harrowing.

It is always interesting when people in your world become gradually aware of your circumstances: co-workers, acquaintances, etc. Truth be told, few people know how to comfortably interact with someone who has cancer. For me, I found that people fell into a few categories. Some people are truly wonderful, kind and supportive right from the get-go. Then there are some people who had heard my situation through others, and boy, are they often awkward! I could tell when someone fell into this category. They tend to say nothing to me, and stare at my boobs as I walk towards them. I remember thinking, "HELLOOOO? they don't look any different yet folks. You can't tell they have cancer in them by staring at them." Ugh, it might as well be high school all over again. Then there are those who are blissfully unaware. I felt bad when one of them would find out and then be all upset as they had to wrap their mind around the news. It is always odd to watch people go through processing the information when you are further along in your own personal acceptance process.

I will say this: life is not fair, cancer is not fair. Cancer doesn't discriminate nor does it care what you have going on in your life. It didn't care that I had a 2 year old at home to raise or a husband whose world would be shattered if something happened to me. It didn't matter to cancer that we had just begun planning to have a second child. In fact, in my specific case, cancer decided that I could NOT have that second child. It pisses me off that cancer had the ability to make that decision for me. It didn't matter to cancer that I had only recently was enjoying the career success I had being working so hard towards since I graduated college. Cancer did not care that we had a family vacation planned for a week that would end up being right in the middle of treatment. And cancer certainly didn't care 8 months later that my mom had been through hell supporting me, and decided to go after her too... Bastard!

Truth be told, a cancer diagnosis is never timed well. Face it, even the most meticulous schedule planners (and I do have a handful of these people in my life, as I am sure you do) couldn't sit down with their smart phone or calendar and say "next spring would be an excellent time for a devastating illness to come my way. I could fit it in nicely then." It just doesn't work that way. Cancer is the rudest party crasher you will ever encounter, especially since it leaves you with a terrible hang over and one heck of a mess to clean up after.

Its devious nature is what makes cancer the worst kind of bully: it's invasive, obviously unwelcome and it's incredibly sneaky. It hits you from behind when you are not looking. It is the true test of mental and physical strength because it seeks to knock you off balance when your back is turned. It doesn't give you time to mentally prepare or practice. It tip-toes up behind you and tries to swallow you whole. And truth be told, it leaves a lasting impression on you no matter what.

Picture this: you are at the beach on a gorgeous summer day. Presumably you have on sunblock because you are mindful of the potential harmful effects of the sun's rays, right? You notice the ocean is calm, and the weather is warm: the perfect combination to take a dip in the ocean. You walk to the water line, breathing in the lovely salt air, feeling content in that moment. You float along peaceful, bobbing gently in the rolling surf. Then suddenly, bam! Without warning, you are hit with a violent wave. It drags you under, shoves water up your nose, and tumbles you head over heels in its fury. As you struggle to determine which end is up, you gag on the salty water, get seaweed in your hair, and sand in your bathing suit. You might even find the top of your bathing suit ripped off, for the world to see (it definitely feels like this once you start to see doctors and everyone wants to take a gander at your "girls"). Once the wave passes, you stand there stunned, fix your suit, coughing and sputtering, wondering what the hell just happened. Eventually, you will regain your composure and recover, but the experience is just downright dreadful. That, my friends, is what it's like to receive a diagnosis of breast cancer! It is nothing short of utterly disorienting and painful.

But this book isn't meant to focus on how much cancer sucks. You certainly don't need me to tell you that. I'm sure you are well aware of that fact. The book is about what you can do to manage the experience a little better and hopefully make your journey a little easier. I found it to be comforting when I knew what to expect. This book is about educating you on breast cancer so as to ready you should you be called into battle. It's about how to arm yourself and it's about how to nurse your wounds (physically and emotionally) as you recover. As traumatic and as horrifying as it can be, the best way to assert your own power over this tormentor is to know your stuff, believe in yourself, stare it down, and if you can, find a way to laugh in its face.

The very first piece of advice I received from another survivor was this: don't let cancer define you. As much as it can be all consuming, especially in the early days, it is not the crux of who you are. Before this, you were many wonderful things. After I hung up the phone with her, I reflected on that thought. It took a great deal of effort to remember that behind that big red flag in my medical chart was a real person. I sat down the night after I was diagnosed, and wrote my very first piece which was designed to remind me of who I was prior to cancer. It was invigorating and necessary to really think through that and realize how much I love me.

I remember early on thinking to myself that I wanted to be a survivor someday. In my mind, they were real life heroes. They had faced unspeakable trials, and came out victorious. I aspired to earning the "right" to wear a survivor t-shirt. Although, I didn't know exactly what the threshold was that would earn me this distinction, but it was something I aimed for. There is no clearly defined finished line where they hand you your survivor medal and you go on your merry way. Somewhere along the line, I realized that I already was one of these brave women.

It's so easy to get lost in your diagnosis, to have it devour you. In my humble opinion, the moment you get your diagnosis and do not drop from the shock is the very moment you become a survivor. The way I see it, all you go through during the process of being diagnosed, deciding on treatment, and then of course treatment itself, are things you survive that are unique and incredibly challenging. On the road to diagnosis, you are squished, stuck with needles, tormented emotionally. If you are still standing after that, you have earned the title of survivor! Others may disagree, and that is ok. We all are entitled to our own interpretations of the word.

Every step along the way requires strength and endurance. We suffer in telling our loved ones the news, knowing we are causing them heartache. I think this was worse for me than knowing myself that I had it. I hated being the cause of sadness to those I love. We undergo the stress of testing. We endure the wait to hear the results of the tests, which is infinitely more torturous than the actual tests themselves. We then are faced with gut wrenching decisions about our health and path forward. Then comes treatment, and everyone knows what a monster that can be. Each of these events is something we survive. So, if you have heard those dreadful words "you have cancer", and didn't drop dead from the shock, then give yourself credit. You too are already a survivor. Wear your shirt or your pink super-hero cape proudly!

Truth be told, a cancer battle is just that: a battle, and when you get the news, once you regain your composure, you will need to suit up. In my experience, I found that it requires a few things. It requires you to find your strength. There are a lot of challenges that you will face. It pushes you mentally and physically. You will get weary. When those days come, it's ok to give yourself rest, just don't stay down too long. A wonderful person once sent me a note saying "be kind to yourself". I cried at this simple message, but realized, she was very right. I was never very good at that and it needed to change. That was hard for me, but I learned that sometimes no matter how strong I wanted to be, I needed to take time to rest and recharge.

Think about it this way, if you hired a personal trainer to get yourself in shape, they will tell you when you are developing a workout plan, it is critical to build in time for your body to rest and recover. Cancer is mental strength training, and a physical endurance challenge. Treat it as you would any workout. Don't give up, but balance out your training appropriately. Take it one day at a time, and expect some down time. This is not the time to test your limits, chemo will do enough of that for you. Listen to your body and go with what it tells you. In the end, you will end up stronger for having rested.

Another component to the fight is maintaining hope. In the middle of my treatment, a wise woman told me, "there is always hope in cancer". By this she means, every day, there are clinical studies going on, and new advancements being discovered.

Treatments that did not exist 10 years ago are now becoming standard of care. Every year, survival rates improve. Hope gives you the drive to fight because it makes you look forward to a bright future. And believe it or not, a bright future is very possible, and often very probable. Educate yourself on the constant, exciting evolution of cancer treatments. Learn how things that were not possible just 10 years ago are available and working today. Believe there is always hope! There are some pretty amazing and relentless scientists out there who are focused on always learning more and advancing care.

Love is also a critical factor in your battle gear. Some days you need to love yourself enough to make tough choices and believe that you are worth going through hell for. Sometimes, you need to focus your love externally, to family and friends, even pets! I can tell you this, there were times when I felt weak, but it was the love for the wonderful people in my world that motivated me to keep going. I couldn't stand the thought of seeing them hurt if I were to quit, so I pushed forward. I had an obligation to them to do the best I could to make this right, and give this fight my everything. And do not forget to let people love you in return. Love begets love and positive energy begets positive energy. It feeds and nourishes your soul. It's critical to learn how to accept help and love during your treatment. You deserve it!

And lastly, you need a sense of humor. My mantra through this ordeal has been: "Cancer is serious enough on its own. It doesn't need me to add to it." A lot of comical things happen along the cancer journey. Laughter makes things a little more manageable. It treats your soul while other things treat your body. Try to make it as light as you can, as you have a heavy enough burden to carry.

Buy yourself a funny wig and wear it out in public at least once! Mine was a short pink bob. Think of the character Frenchie in Grease. That was the look I was sporting. Admittedly, I only had the guts to wear it around the time of Halloween. There I was, at my son's preschool, all pinked out. Most of the moms knew what was going on and I think appreciated my ability to keep the situation light. My brother wanted me to go with the curly clown wig, but I wimped out. Somehow, Frenchie, I was ok with, but Clarabell the clown, not so much!

3. TESTS AND DECISION-MAKING

It's hard to say what is worse: knowing you have cancer, or waiting for various test results once you are in the throes of it all. I was lucky. The process of getting diagnosed was pretty quick for me. There was a flurry of activity in the span of a few hours, but I was lucky. I had my answer within 24 hours. I was impressed with the breast center's turnaround time. Unfortunately, that experience taught me that my world can change in the blink of an eye. I now know that a test can yield unexpected and life-altering results, I instantly dreaded the thought of every test, and tormented myself during the time spent in no woman's land waiting for the results. It's simply amazing how quickly the mind can run away with itself in the absence of information.

I do think the period of waiting for answers is more stressful than knowing. At least when you know, you can plan your next steps. When you are waiting, there's nothing that you can do but wait, and if you are like me, you will likely obsess and drive yourself crazy in the meantime. Let me tell you, feeling helpless and impatient is inevitable, and it's crappy. Nothing gets you more in tune with your inner control freak than a journey through cancer. I really thought I was easy-going, and low-stress.

Wrong-o! I learned I am quite the opposite, at least when it comes to my health. I channeled my inner control-freak extraordinaire.

If you are like me and have never had a serious health issue before breast cancer, you might be shocked at the sheer volume of tests that are coming your way. You will either feel like a pin cushion or a lab rat (or both) by the time you are done with this experience. It gets very tiresome, but there is no getting around it. It's vital information that you need in order to know which path to take going forward.

If you have been diagnosed, there is a good chance you have already had a mammogram, ultrasound, biopsy and possibly even an MRI. By the way, MRIs are torture. They slide you into this tiny tube, and then for about a half hour, you are engulfed in the most atrocious noise. I came out with a migraine! I complained to my doctor about it, and he told me he cried the whole time through his first MRI. You might want to take a preemptive strike of Tylenol and anti-anxiety meds before you go into the torture tube. If they discover tumor cells in the lymph nodes, then you are likely in for a whole other battery of tests to be sure that the disease hasn't set up camp anywhere else. It is not uncommon to have a bone scan, a pet scan, an MRI or a ct scan shortly after being diagnosed.

In order to do each of these tests, you will be injected with or have to consume some sort of tracer or contrast. Then they put you in these monstrous machines and scan away looking for uptake of the tracers. Basically, each of these tracers tags a different type of anomaly in the body, and the machines can tell if there is a possible malignancy. Breast cancer metastasizes (spreads) to places like the lungs, liver, bones or brain. The course of treatment is dictated by not only the type of tumor, but also where it is present.

These tests definitely fall into the category of "who on earth figured this stuff out?" Throughout this whole process, I really developed a new appreciation for science as it baffles me that people are able to determine that a random concoction would cling to cancer cells in the bones and make it light up in a scan. I found it fascinating and so crazy! It made me want to go out and hug a nerd!

Going through the actual tests themselves really isn't too bad. It's the time that comes between getting dressed and walking out of the hospital, and waiting for that phone call that is pure hell. The sad part is, the people who work at hospitals of course take their jobs seriously, but might not put the same urgency on finalizing your results as you would. There have been times where I know the report had been read, but the final verdict hadn't been presented to my doctor. Talk about infuriating! If you are like me, you will convince yourself of the most unlikely, worst-case scenarios until you hear otherwise. When that phone rings, your heart will stop and you will want to throw up. They should really give out barf bags upon your diagnosis.

But as emotionally challenging as tests can be, they are necessary. It's important to know what's going on inside of you so you can take the best course of action for your unique set of circumstances. The sad reality is that cancer is so sneaky, you can't always go by symptoms to determine where it is present or what it's doing in your body. Often times, symptoms (aside from breast lumps) don't manifest until later stages with cancer. So the testing is about getting all your facts to help you make decisions based on every piece of applicable information. The more you know, the more you can tailor your treatment plan to what is most effective for a profile like yours. Knowledge is power, and that is no less true in the world of cancer.

It is so important to remember that every single patient and every single incidence of cancer is unique. So too are the decisions that each individual must make. It's human nature to look to others for validation of our choices, especially choices that have such serious implications, but in this case, we really need to recognize that each person's cancer is different. Each patient needs to work with their medical team to determine what is best for them, and it is more than ok to recognize that what works for someone else may not work for you. There are standards of care based on each person's tumor pathology and stage, but even those are not set in stone.

The best thing a patient can do is arm themselves with information and make thoughtful, independent decisions that resonate with their own heart. Each patient has to live their own life and has to be able to sleep at night knowing they made the best decisions they could regarding their health. This can be an incredibly daunting task at a time when your brain is numb, and particularly challenging if you are like me and have no medical background. Not only do you have to make intense decisions, you have to do it based on information that might sound like a foreign language to you!

For anyone going through this, your life will become one big appointment calendar for quite a while. This was hard for me to adjust to considering I was tended to see a doctor no more than two times per year on average. If you work, I personally recommend making sure that your colleagues know what is going on. You will need to focus on your health and that will require a lot of time and flexibility. Your priorities will shift as a result of this, at least while you are going through testing and treatment, and they need to know that. I find that the more people know, the more support you will receive.

There is a lot of information that will play into determining what the appropriate care is for you. I want to reiterate (again) that each patient is different and has a unique cancer pathology. That profile determines what the options are for an appropriate treatment plan. It could be any combination of surgery, chemotherapy, radiation, and hormonal therapy and additional medical treatment. Treatment will consume a good portion of your time in the coming months. It's so critical for you to be actively involved in the decision making process. Even though there are typical protocols for each profile, you still will have decisions to make. Your body is going to go through a lot, and it's essential that you are aware, understand and are comfortable with what is going to happen to you. After all, it is your body, no one else's. You have to live with it all.

Before you start your whirlwind of appointments, you might want to treat yourself to a cute tote bag/large purse. You are going to want to bring a notebook with you to your appointments and buy yourself an expandable file folder because you will accumulate a lot of paper in the coming months. So why not carry those babies around in style. Just because you have breast cancer doesn't mean that you can't still be trendy.

You will quickly be buried under mountains of forms, information sheets, contact information, test results and medical bills. It will be difficult to keep track of all of the paper, but each one is important. Keep good records and keep your paperwork straight. It is very easy to let that get away from you, but your life will be much easier if you take control and develop a system for maintaining your records. Unfortunately, at a time when it feels like there are things coming at you from every direction, and it is hard to keep up, more than ever, you need to get organized, and for those of you who know me personally, I am sure you are all having a good chuckle over me saying this: I am quite possibly the least organized person in the world. Many of you are familiar with my filing system: i.e. "the pile o' crap".

It might also be helpful for you to learn the titles of all of the medical professionals that you will soon be spending an excessive amount of time with. This is a whole new team you will be working with, with new fancy titles and job descriptions. It took me a while to get straight in my own mind who did what, so now that I have it finally figured out, I will pass it along to you.

The first people you will likely encounter are the technicians. They are usually the ones who are performing your mammos, ultrasounds, MRIs, assisting in biopsies, etc. They are the people who are there in the very beginning to welcome you to this crazy place. Just don't expect them to give you answers. Even though they probably have them, they are usually are not allowed to tell you. But watch their faces, their expressions might tell you what you need to know (just beware of the "oh shit" face as I mentioned earlier).

The information the techs gather is then interpreted and shared with you by a Radiologist, who is a medical doctor who specializes in reviewing the scans and preparing the official results. You will probably feel somewhat attached to this person, but don't get too comfortable. You will likely not hang out with them once you are diagnosed, except for maybe when you do follow up tests. I was bummed at that fact because since she was the first doctor to see me in this new world, I wanted to cling to her for dear life out of fear. She was so nice and compassionate.

The next member of your team is very important one: your breast surgeon. I remember hearing early on that the most critical doctor to select is your surgeon. You want someone who is precise, experienced, and thorough. Their job is to get the cancer out of you! So they need to be on the top of their game when in surgery. No easy feat when they can't see every cell that is in there. You might potentially need a reconstructive surgeon to partner with your breast surgeon depending on the type of surgery you have. Obviously, you want a good one here too because they are the ones responsible for making you look pretty after the fact. If you can find out who all the nurses go to for their tummy tucks, etc. then that's usually a good sign of their skills and reputation!

You will also need a medical oncologist. This is your long-term partner. He or she will basically be your case manager and set your overall treatment and follow-up plan. They will be the one who devise your chemo plan if one is necessary, and who will basically be your main go-to doctor. You will likely spend more time with this doctor than any other. When we get to the chemo chapter, I will talk more about what you need to consider when selecting your medical oncologist.

If you elect to have radiation therapy, you also will have a radiation oncologist who will design that part of your treatment plan and administer that course. Your radiation oncologist is not to be confused with a radiologist. Trust me, it took me a while to keep those two straight. Most cancer patients struggle with this one. I find this is the most common point of confusion for people when they are talking about their medical team.

When you are just starting off, I highly recommend going for multiple opinions with all of the doctors. This will allow you to feel hopefully more comfortable with the once you choose to go with for your treatment. Even if they end up telling you the same thing, it will be helpful. Think of it as sports try-outs, where you are the coach. You want to be sure you pick the players for your team that impress you the most. You need to feel confident that the doctors you are meeting with are worthy of having the honor of treating you.

Remember that you are special, and you deserve the best of care. Don't settle for less than that, and don't worry about hurting a doctor's feelings by asking questions or deciding they are not the right fit for you. This is not a time to be polite. It's a time to be assertive and self-focused! Make sure you are comfortable with each of member of your team, and remember that you are the boss. They need to work up to your expectations, and if they don't, pull a "Donald Trump" and fire them! There are tons of excellent doctors around and you don't need to settle. These doctors hold your life in their hands, be sure they earn that privilege.

It is so important in those early stages of diagnosis to assign someone to be your advocate. This is someone who can come to your doctor's appointment and be a second set of ears for you. They can help you remember details and prompt you with what questions you should be asking. It doesn't matter who that person is, as long as they have a clear mind and can recall and translate the details of the endless string of medical appointments. Trust me, these interactions will start to blend after a while and it will get hard to keep the details straight. Don't rely solely on your brain to keep this information. Even if you had a photographic memory before, you still will have a hard time retaining and deciphering facts. It's simply too much information. After a while, all that scientific mumbo jumbo starts to ooze out of your ears if you are not careful.

I appointed my sister-in-law and mother to the challenging task of helping me keep track of it all in the early days. My brain was like a saturated sponge and simply could not absorb much more information. If I had to go it alone, I am certain I would have missed about seventy-five percent of what was said. Everything is so confusing and overwhelming in the early days, it's so hard to keep your facts straight and focus. As I mentioned earlier, having little medical background, I was thrust into this horrid new world where I did not know the language. I was about to get the crash course of a lifetime. This was worse than any accelerated program I took during my college or post-graduate career. That is for certain.

Also, I cannot stress this enough: learn to go with your gut. You will need and deserve to be an active part of your decision making team. Do not allow doctors to simply dictate your treatment plan without understanding it yourself. It is perfectly ok to ask "why?" or "why not" when presented with options. Do your research, talk to others who have been through it, even if that is through breast cancer websites, but please, if you go online ONLY stick to reputable sites, like www.komen.org or www.cancer.org. There is too much crap out there that will only scare you and may not even be remotely applicable to your situation. Learn about your diagnosis, your body and the treatment options. Learn about the risks associated with the treatment plans. It's critical that you understand what is being proposed and why it's the best course for you. It will help you to understand what to expect, and it will make you feel empowered. Navigating your way through this foreign territory takes a lot of time, energy, attention and the aptitude to learn a whole lot of new information.

It is very empowering to educate yourself and actively participate in the decision-making process. I remember someone reminding me, "you have spent your whole life making quality decisions for yourself. What makes you think you can't still make good decisions now? You can. Cancer doesn't change that." Harness that fact in your situation too. Take ownership of your decisions as it will help you emotionally as well. It will help you reclaim the sense of control that you likely feel was stolen by cancer.

Doctors will discuss your options with you and often are very careful to stress that you have choices to make. Many times, they try to stay not to push to fervently in one direction or another, especially before they have established a relationship with you. I always found it helpful to ask the doctors the following: "Doctor, I understand I have options, but tell me what you would recommend to me if I were your daughter or wife." I found that they were honest in their reply, and that helped me to confidently choose what path I would take going forward.

In my first few weeks, I saw three surgeons to discuss next steps and basically to decide who I was going to trust with my life. No pressure! Two of them had very similar recommendations, and I believe that I would have been fine with either one of them. The third was absolutely technically competent, but didn't seem to understand my needs as a patient or a woman as well as the other two did. I felt pressured towards surgical options that I didn't feel was appropriate for my lifestyle. Given that, I chose one of the other surgeons: the one that seemed the best fit for me, not just by her skills, but by her understanding of me as an individual. That was so important for me to establish trust that she had my best interests at heart.

One other option you might want to consider is participation in a clinical research study. Studies are happening every day in every aspect of treatment. Not all doctors participate in studies, but you might want to ask what ones are happening currently. Especially with breast cancer, there is always research going on to test different protocols, new technology, assess quality of life issues for different treatment options, etc. You might find this an interesting opportunity. It might provide you with the chance to be on the cutting edge of treatment.

When you participate in the studies, you also have all medical bills related to that study covered by whoever is running it. This can be appealing in this day and age when healthcare coverage is such a disaster. There's also the upside of knowing you are helping future cancer survivors by helping them to learn more about our disease. This is a pretty exciting experience to be a part of.

However, of course, the point of doing a study is to learn about these new treatment options. With that, comes inherent risk of the unknown. That may very well be a valid turnoff for some women. Either way, it's worth exploring to determine if it may be an option for you. I wish I had been aware of some studies that went on while I was getting treated. I didn't know they were an option, and would have liked the opportunity to have considered them. My mother was able to learn from my experience, and chose to participate in a radiation therapy study. She was extra pleased because she got selected for the group that was in treatment for a shorter time frame, which meant she finished treatment quicker. Who doesn't want this nonsense behind them as quickly as possible?

Anyone who knew me when I was "Nicole before cancer" or "NBC" for short, knew that I was not a fan of confrontation and I felt terrible rejecting someone or saying anything that might hurt someone's feelings. Well, "Nicole with cancer" is a different broad all together. I had to learn rather quickly to not be so nice, and just be genuine, honest and assertive. I did need reminders that it so ok to do this along the way. As a patient, you can't put your life in someone else's hands if you are not confident that they are going to do what is best for you. Sometimes, this even means changing doctors midstream. (Yes, I did this half way through chemo, if you can believe it). You are an individual, different than anyone else in this world. Your life, your body, and your health are unique to you and only you. As such, you need to have a medical team that recognizes this and treats you like the rock-star that you are.

I am only going to say this once, and it might sounds like a taboo suggestion, but here goes nothing. When you get diagnosed with something like cancer, you have the right to be selfish. GASP! I said it, and in public, no less! I remember talking to one of my friends right after learning the news, and I said to her "who will take care of everyone while I am sick?" That truly was a huge concern for me. She calmly said, "We will take care of each other and for once, it's time for you to let us take care of you". For me, as for most breast cancer survivors, this was a huge adjustment.

Your job for the next few months is to get through treatment as uneventfully as possible, and to surround yourself with the best medical professionals and emotional support you need to manage through this trying journey. Focus on yourself for a change. Do what is right for you. Here's a way you might be able to reframe what I just said that might make you feel better about it. If you are selfish now, you can go back to spoiling those you love when this is all over.

In a world where I was conditioned to be considerate of others feelings often before my own; in a world where I do believe that if you have nothing nice to say, you should say nothing at all; in a world where I have often compromised what I would like for someone else's happiness, I say this: in times like this, you just have to put yourself and your health first. Based on the role we women often play in society, it's natural for us to put our needs last. That's often who we are at our core. Sad, but true. But when you are battling a major illness, the best thing you can do is to make yourself a priority. I had expectations of myself and what I was used to doing, and others did as well. That was a shift for a lot of people. Some people had a hard time accepting "no" from me. But eventually, I learned that I have to put my health before someone else's feelings, including doctors and their staff. You can do it politely, but you will need to learn to stand up for yourself, no matter how intimidating that might feel. Say what you need to say. Ask what you need to ask. Do what you need to do. Do not be shy. Now is not the time to be timid!

So let's recap. Educate yourself. Explore your options. Trust your gut. Do not be afraid to ask questions. Be your own boss, and make your medical team be accountable to your needs and wants. Bring someone with you to all appointments as a second set of ears. You will have major decisions to make about your body and your care in the early days when your brain is still fuzzy from shock. It might feel like trying to run a mile when your foot is asleep. It's awkward and painful, but you have to do it. This is why having an extra set of ears with you in your appointments, as well as a note pad will come in handy. It will become difficult to sort through all of the information and recommendation alone. These decisions will be some of the most important ones you will ever make. You want to be able to look back at this time when it's all done and have no regrets.

4. YOUR SOUL NEEDS CARE TOO

There is a component of treatment that is often overlooked and underestimated. Most doctors do an outstanding job treating your body, but honestly, there is so much more damage that a breast cancer diagnosis then what a scalpel or an iv infusion can fix. Cancer shakes you to the core. It's just a fact. Your mind, heart and soul are also critically affected by this experience. If you ignore them, you will likely struggle for a long time. And truth be told, your mental health and your physical health are closely linked. Wellness seems to be most effective when it comes from a comprehensive approach, aligning all that is part of you to head in the same positive, healthy direction. It's critical to get harmony within and to recognize that it may take some effort for that to happen. And remember, what you are encountering is not your garden-variety stress. This is heavy-duty stuff! Treat it appropriately.

During my very first visit with my oncologist, she stressed the importance of this. She gave me a homework assignment to attend sessions at a local support group. At first, I hesitated. I didn't think I needed it. It made me feel self-conscious and afraid. I think this was partially due to the denial I had that the diagnosis I was experiencing was traumatic and a pretty big deal. I promised her I would consider it, and I got over my initial hesitation and started attending programs at the Cancer Support Community. Once I did, I was hooked. I quickly became a believer that the mind and soul have a huge role in the recovery process. There was no denying the impact of the groups and sessions I attended. They soothed my soul, much in the way Zofran soothed my nausea.

Let's face it, not only is the diagnosis traumatic, but the treatments that follow can be as well. We are human, and no matter how strong we are, we are affected by our experiences. Cancer is no exception to that rule. As much as we know the importance of treatments, enduring the side effects can be demoralizing. So what people don't often expect is the emotional side effects that come along with treatment. Everyone copes and manages the emotions in different ways, so it is important to find a strategy that works for you. I will say this though, burying the emotions and ignoring the fact that they exist is probably not the most effective approach. They will only come and find their way to the surface at some point. But I am no expert. I am just someone who has lived it and watched others as well.

One key coping technique is for you to find survivors who can serve as beacons of hope and pillars of support for you. Talking with survivors can provide you with so many benefits. They will show you that your journey, albeit unpleasant, is doable. They also will remind you that despite the fact that it feels so isolating, you are not alone in this process. So many women have taken this trip before you. I cannot tell you how therapeutic this can be to connect with these ladies. The very morning after I got diagnosed and realized it wasn't a bad dream, I called a survivor who was near and dear to my heart. She told me in no uncertain terms this sucks, but you can do this. And you know what? I believed her because she was 8 years out. That was my first moment of calm. Having other survivors as resources is invaluable. It provides you with a source of optimism and comfort as you see women living normal lives after walking in your shoes. They also can give you perspective and suggestions that you will not be able to get from someone who has not been through this, including doctors.

Don't hesitate to reach out if you know survivors. Most are ready, willing and able to help a sister. Even if they were very private about their own experience, I have found they are willing to be open and helpful to those who get diagnosed after them. So many woman feel a special calling to help others because they know that lonely feeling that can come with cancer. It does our hearts good to be of comfort and support to someone because we know how that helped us. You also might be surprised when you get diagnosed how many people you know are affected and you were unaware. Some survivors are loud and bold in their journey (such as yours truly), but some do it privately, and do not tell those around them. Often times, you learn of these people only after you have been diagnosed.

If you do not yet have any of these amazing women in your life, there are many ways to find them. You can find them online. Do searches for cancer support message boards. There are plenty of breast cancer sites that have this feature and they can be such a wonderful resource. There are some that target special needs, they can focus on surgery options, other treatment options, different cancer profiles, even young survivorship (which has its own set of challenges). You will find members are willing to share and support you by answering questions and letting you know what their experience has been. Some of the steps along your journey may seem so very strange and unnerving to you, until you realize how common place they are. There is a sense of relief that this happens to people, and they get through it.

There are also several wonderful support services available out there that are available to you at no cost. Many cancer treatment centers offer free programs to patients and their families. The Cancer Support Community and Gilda's Club are two tremendous organizations. The Cancer Support Community was the group my doctor recommended to me at that first appointment, and it has been so very critical to my experience. I still attend programs and find them to be helpful each and every time. I have attended workshops, seminars, support groups and individual counseling. I am convinced that my individual counselor has a magic wand. It is without fail that when I am done with a conversation with her, I feel stronger, more hopeful and more empowered. I find that I cannot go more than a month without talking to her. I have learned so much from the other community members and from their staff. They have made my journey so much easier by sharing ideas, suggestions and experiences. My soul always felt soothed when I walk out of those doors. It's like aloe for the soul. When I go too long in between sessions, I find my emotions getting out of whack, and I struggle much more. Those struggles bleed into other parts of my life, so it's important to keep them in check.

Believe it or not, I even met several survivors doing event walks for breast cancer charities. Walks can be incredibly life-affirming and emotional. I cannot tell you how touched I was at my very first walk, when my tell-tale bald head was not well hidden under a light ski cap. I was clearly a rookie in the world of breast cancer. I was terribly self-conscious and almost embarrassed. Then something wonderful happened: several long-term survivors reached out to me and offered me words of encouragement and hugs. These were women who didn't know me, they just understood that I was new to their world. And they knew that in that moment, what I needed most was to hear that I too would be ok. I never saw them again, but in that moment, they knew that I needed hope and they provided it. I thank God for those ladies that day. They were angels in the moment when I needed them the most.

I am sure you already know that cancer survivors are strong and inspiring. That's the image that is out there in the world. However, did you know that they are hilarious, helpful, and supportive? They will make you laugh because if you look hard enough, there are some pretty funny elements to this crazy experience. You just have to have an open mind. They also often have little tolerance for nonsense because a diagnosis like this puts everything in perspective. The petty things become less important. It strips away your ability to mire in too much nonsense. Survivors are often honest and open. They have dealt with awkward side effects and often have good tips on how to manage them. They will tell you things that no doctor will tell you. They will help you when you inevitably think to yourself "Oh my God! Is this normal?" They are not a substitute for your doctor, but rather they supplement the information you are gaining from your medical team. For example, I cannot tell you how relieved I was to find out that craving Chinese food is a common occurrence during chemo! Who knew? Survivors, that's who! So I wholeheartedly say find them and surround yourself with them. They will fill your heart with joy, understanding and camaraderie.

In addition to survivors, you will have your co-survivors: the people in your old world who walk this new journey with you. They are the ones who shared your life with you before cancer turned it upside down. Co-survivors are as traumatized as you are by your diagnosis. They are often the ones you think of first and dread telling the minute you get that call. They are the ones who know all of the wonderful things that you are besides cancer.

Every co-survivor of them will handle your disease differently, just as every survivor handles it differently. Some might rally around you, bold and loud. Some will discreetly find ways to support you. Some may proudly wear a bracelet with your name on it or a pink ribbon on their shirt. Some will simply remember you in their daily prayers. Some will want to crawl into a hole, hide and pretend like the whole things is a bad dream. The pain may just be more than they can bear. Try to remember that they too are struggling. It is so very difficult to watch someone you love go through a cancer battle. For some, it may even be harder than if they were going through it themselves. Most of them will feel helpless at one time or another. Not knowing what to do can only perpetuate that feeling. There is nothing worse than feeling helpless.

As a patient and survivor, it's so important to learn how to vocalize your thoughts and feelings, whether that be to a doctor, a therapist or a co-survivor. For a long time, we often try to mask it, and say everything is just fine. We are often used to being strong for others, and we try to carry that into cancer. But the truth is, some days, things are not fine and we need extra support. It can be hard to break away from trying to protect those that we love. We basically need to check the stubborn pride at the door, and realize that they are waiting to take their cues from us. Sometimes the best thing we can do for them and for us is to open up and let them in. They often want to be a part of supporting you and helping you shoulder the burden. It's often a refreshing feeling for all involved when we stop protecting each other and we become honest. It's an experience that is best conquered when be shared. Until you can learn how to do that, you will likely feel extremely lonely, and that will not help your state of mind.

Allow yourself and others to have emotional days. They are a normal, cathartic part of the healing process. As much as we sometimes want to be rock strong all of the time, it's just not realistic. We are human. It's ok to be scared. It's ok to be angry. It's ok to be sad. It's ok to be frustrated. What's not ok is to stay that way permanently. Experience the emotions. Share them with others if that helps. Let them pass through you, like bubbles rising up in a glass of seltzer water. Let them live their life, and then move on from them. If you release them, even if it's slowly, you will heal from them. If you find that you are unable to manage the emotions and they are interfering with your ability to function, seek professional help. There are some outstanding social workers, therapists, psychologists and psychiatrists who specialize in working with oncology patients. Think of it this way, if you seek them out, you are helping the economy by giving them work to do. Really, it's a win-win.

Anger is a pretty common emotion that survivors will encounter. I can't lie, it really ticked me off that this came into my life and I had no control over it. I was so aggravated at cancer for blindsiding me. I was mad at it for interfering with my life. It affected every aspect of my life in some way and that bothered me. There were times when I was just plain mad that I got picked to have this disease. I didn't ask for it. I know no one does, but that fact doesn't make it feel any less unfair when it happens to you. Having been a pretty driven person throughout my life, having something like cancer tell me I couldn't do something that I wanted, or make me physically unable to care for my child, or causing me to miss a family event just infuriated me. There were times when I really resented the disease for the control it exerted over me at times.

There was a sense of unfairness that came with getting sick. I felt like I didn't deserve this. Of course, the truth is, no one ever deserves to get it. I almost wish there was such a thing as karma when it came to cancer. But it doesn't work that way. Sadly, the likes of Hitler and Osama bin Laden did not get cancer. Instead, good people sometimes get it. The truth is, even though it might feel like it, cancer is not a punishment. It's just a disease that happens. There isn't much we can do to control whether or not we get it. Of course, there are some lifestyle choices that can help mitigate the risks, even those are not a certain guarantee against it.

There were other times that I just felt sad and depressed. It was a very helpless feeling when there was no one who could tell me where my cancer came from or what I could have done differently. It was discouraging to me because I wanted so badly to do everything I could to prevent it from ever coming back. But since I didn't know what caused it, I could only do the best I could and attempt to live a healthy life style and hope for the best. Akin to this was the resentment of those who blatantly abused their bodies. It was frustrating to see people making choices that were harmful to themselves, when I wasn't given a choice. I made healthy choices and they didn't guarantee me anything. I also was sad because there were times when the disease made me feel defective. I tried to focus on the mantra that everything happens for a reason and turn my illness into an opportunity to make positive impact as a result but there were days when that was really hard.

Sometimes, I felt confident and strong. For whatever reason, I got this awful disease, and I had to deal with some pretty brutal stuff to treat it. That's kind of a big deal, and sometimes, we as survivors don't give ourselves enough credit for the challenges we face on a regular basis. Every once in a while, I would try to pause and reflect on that. I had the disease, I treated it with everything I could, and I kept moving forward. I worked hard to make the world better for me having had cancer. I do believe have made a small dent. One never knows what will pop up in the future, but none the less, I can honestly say I gave it my all against some pretty challenging circumstances, and for that I am proud.

And of course there were times when I felt scared. Unfortunately that was more often than not, and sadly, it still happens fairly regularly. Cancer and fear are pretty constant companions. I think fear is the most intense and most underestimated emotional side effect of this disease. It's incredibly impactful. Once you get a diagnosis of cancer, you feel horribly vulnerable. It's a terrible feeling. I remember early on hearing that once people were diagnosed, they dreaded doctor's visits. I didn't grasp why that was until I experienced it for myself. Up until this point, doctors were innocuous. Before cancer, nothing that ever happened at a doctor's appointment was grossly life changing or shocking. But life is a series of learning experiences strung together, and so once you get your diagnosis, you learn that your life can change drastically and instantaneously. That is just daunting! Appointments then start to take on way more importance and there for drum up some hefty anxiety. Cancer tends to breed its own brand of post-traumatic stress!

There have even been times when I feel like all of this is just a dream. It doesn't seem real to me. Granted it has lasted a lot longer than most dreams do, but it's quite surreal. No one ever expects to be a cancer survivor, so when you find yourself in the middle of it, it can be very disorienting. There are times when I stop and wonder how I got to this place in my life. I sometimes don't recognize my own self or the situation around me. But there is nothing I can do to change what has happened, so I plod forward.

One of the best techniques for managing emotion during my journey has been writing. I started a blog the very day after I received my diagnosis. That blog was the springboard into my newfound medium. It was the predecessor of this book. It was one of the best forms of therapy for me. It was a great catharsis. Many nights, I was unable to sleep until I wrote out what was rattling around in my mind. I often focused on positive, uplifting themes, partially for me, and partially as a way of supporting my co-survivors to try to help them understand what I was going through. I used the blog as my rally point. I was fortunate to receive such amazing encouragement from my readers on my writings. That, in turn, fostered the desire to write and share my experiences with a broader audience: to anyone who could potentially learn and be positively affected by my words.

While I realize that public sharing of emotion in this day and age is somewhat common place with all of the social networking technology out there, I recognize that not everyone is comfortable putting their experience with cancer on display. There are other ways to use creative outlets in more private forms. For example, personal journaling has a very similar effect to the blogging for many people. In some ways, you might find this to be more comfortable because you can be honest about your experiences without fear of judgment or causing distress to others.

For me, I do 90 percent of my writing in a public fashion, but there is another 10 percent that is strictly private. They may be too intense, emotional or painful to share with others, even my super emotional and supportive family. I consider these the "lost blogs" and they are solely for my own personal need and they are kept in a serenity journal. One woman told me she privately journaled through her experience, she shared her writings with no one and when she was done with treatment and felt ready, she burned those books as a way to release those emotion. I found that to be a beautiful method of healing and letting go of the past.

Many also find other creative avenues. Crocheting, knitting, pottery, scrapbooking, jewelry-making are just a few other ways to channel all the energy or angst that is inside you. Physical outlets are also great coping mechanisms. For example, there are special yoga and strength training classes designed for cancer patients that are just a true blessing for some. I personally benefitted tremendously from guided imagery and mediation. I have done sessions in person at the Cancer Support Community and have found some online that I would do at home as well. I find them to be simply soothing and a highly effective way to take the edge off the stress. There were many nights where I would not have slept at all if it wasn't for the blogging and the guided imagery to distract my mind from of the stress.

For me, being informed was substantially empowering. I learned to select my sources carefully, because there is an overabundance of information that might not necessarily be relevant. Make a rule for yourself that if you choose to research online, you will only view information from reputable sources. Also, seeking out professionally hosted seminars on nutrition, coping strategies, and just general breast cancer information sessions have been tremendously valuable to me.

One of the most frustrating things about cancer is the fact that there are so many things that we cannot control with it. However, if we inform ourselves, there certainly are some things that we can do to mitigate risks. Knowledge is power. All it takes is arming ourselves with reliable, research-backed information, and putting that information to good use in our lives. One of the benefits of cancer is that if you utilize your information well, you can end up living a much healthier lifestyle that can make a difference in your quality of life and general health. Is it a guarantee that cancer will never return? Unfortunately not, but at least it helps you to give you some peace of mind that you have done the best you can for your health.

I am a huge believer of religious freedom. Given that, I know there is a very wide range of beliefs out there. I know there are plenty of good people who do not have belief in any religion or deity or who do not have an affinity for prayer. For those who do, however, I would suggest that prayer is helpful. If you are a person of faith, this experience will certainly affect the very foundation of your belief system. Whether it does so positively or negatively is a purely individual experience.

For me, it enhanced my faith in many ways, but I would be lying if I said it didn't shake it as well. Like anyone, I have my times when I just couldn't help but wonder why I had been chosen to bear this cross, why anyone is chosen for it for that matter. I spent a lot of time in prayer and reflection trying to gain the best understanding I could. My prayers were varied depending on the circumstances at the time. I prayed to Saint Peregrine, to Our Lady of Mount Carmel, and of course just to God. I reacquainted myself with my bible. And I have to admit, I chuckled when I learned that my smart phone had a free bible app on it. Yes, I downloaded it, and I love it! I swear they have an app for everything these days!

As much as I wanted to turn this challenge into an opportunity for goodness, I am human. This was the hardest experience of my life. I am pretty sure the worst part of it was the fear and lack of control that comes with a cancer diagnosis. Having a solid faith foundation helped, but there were some times when truth be told, even strong faith wasn't enough to mitigate the internal struggles for me. As much as I wanted to live by faith and not fear, it was so very hard. Fear seeks to overwhelm faith, and does a pretty darn good job sometimes.

While I will never quite comprehend why this disease exists, I do believe that since I got it, it's my obligation to seek unique opportunities for me to give back that would not have manifested if it were not for breast cancer. Perhaps one is to make women aware that breast cancer can happen to young women like myself who have no family history. As I have said before, to save another woman's life by prompting them to detect their cancer early is truly the greatest gift to me. Perhaps it is to become a tremendous fundraiser to help with support and research for other patients. Perhaps it's to be an advocate for others who feel they cannot find their voice. Perhaps it is to remind people who have any kind of struggle in their life that they can win, if they just push through the hard times and keep their chin up. These struggles don't have to be cancer. They could be any medical issue, they could be depression, alcoholism, unemployment, an abusive environment or anything troublesome. It could even just be coping with the ups and downs of everyday life.

Regardless of what the struggle is, perhaps my message to the world is that there is always hope and that no matter how overwhelming your challenges maybe, perseverance is so critical to being victorious. And even if we don't exactly get the exact results we hope for, if we hold our heads high and fight our battles with dignity, then we should be proud.

The bottom line is this: the worst thing you can do for yourself is to do nothing. Being inactive, physically or mentally is a recipe for disaster. First off, it's just not good for your body in general. But besides that, it will create hopeless, and might cause you to obsess on every aspect of cancer, and that is just not healthy. As they say, idle hands are the devil's playground, idle minds and bodies are as well. They just don't get you anywhere good. Staying home all the time and having too much time to think is purely detrimental to your healing process. So find something to do, even if it's wrong (just don't do anything illegal!).

I know that while undergoing treatment, it's tough to get up and go sometimes, but it's critical to find those distractions. Keeping that mind busy, and thinking about non-cancerous things are so helpful. You will be amazed when little by little, other thoughts occupy your mind besides the "Big C". It feels pretty wonderful when you allow your mind to delve outside of that cancer realm and think about something else. It reminds you that you are so much more than your diagnosis.

Each patient needs to reflect on what it is they would like to make of the challenges that come their way in life. There is no denying that taking trauma in life and converting it to a positive requires great effort when you are facing something troubling. Sometimes, it just feels easier to give in to the stress and aggravation and let them consume you. However, the rewards of turning a negative into a positive can be life changing, not only for you, but for those whose life you touch by your actions.

On the flip side of survivor stories, there is the risk of hearing horror stories. In our society, everyone loves a horror story. And unfortunately, in the realm of cancer (perhaps more than any other health issue), there are plenty of these to go around. If you find that someone is telling you a story about a cancer patient they know that has an unpleasant circumstance involved, and if you find that this freaks you out, say so! At first, I would politely listen to the stories, and then go have a panic attack somewhere hidden from view. These people mean no harm, but the truth is, they may be inadvertently messing with your mind. If you find a story going down a path that you know is going to get those wheels in your mind turning in an unpleasant direction, tell them politely that it doesn't help you to hear such stories, and change the subject or run for the hills.

Just as positive stories breed hope and positive feelings, negative stories breed fear and negative feelings. You have every right to stop someone from discussion something that is unnecessarily damaging to you. They likely don't even realize the impact this has on you unless you tell them. It will not do you any good to stress out over something that happened to someone else. Think of your mind as a garden: you want your fruits, veggies and flowers to grow there. Don't allow the weeds to soak up any of the nutrition in the soil that is meant for good flora. Pluck that crap right out and let your garden flourish.

And honestly, when all else fails, if you try all of the tactics listed above, and you still are struggling, that is perfectly ok. That's why they make anti-anxiety medications. Talk to your doctor about what options you might have as far as prescription drugs to help manage your situation. They really might be what you need. Don't feel awkward about it. Isn't that what this stuff is made for? Why not use it? It might only need to be a temporary solution to get you through an incredibly rough patch. Don't underestimate the trauma you are experiencing. Give cancer its due props, and then manage it accordingly. Use whatever is necessary to tame that beast! If it gives you any comfort to know, I have taken them under my doctor's care from time to time. There have been times for me when the fear was just unmanageable without medical assistance. I am ok admitting that so that others can feel comfortable seeking that option if it is something that they think they need.

5. SURGICAL CONSIDERATIONS

Before I get into the sensitive subject matter of surgery, I want to acknowledge that every patient has a different surgical approach that is appropriate to them. There are so many options: lumpectomy versus mastectomy; reconstruction versus not. If reconstruction is elected, there are many of methods you can use. When deciding what works for you, you and your doctor will consider several factors: your tumor profile, your body image, your lifestyle, your age, your overall health status (you know, aside from this cancer thing you got going on). For this part of the process, you will need to see a breast surgeon, and if you opt for any form of reconstruction, you will need a reconstructive surgeon. In many cases, they are two separate specialties although some surgeons will do both parts of the job. I bet you never thought you would be seeing a plastic surgeon about a boob job, did ya? I sure as hell didn't. Ah, the ironies of life!

Many women opt for a lumpectomy. Depending on the type of tumor, a lumpectomy can be equally effective as a mastectomy. Essentially, a lumpectomy is a more targeted/less invasive surgery. The doctor goes in and removes the known malignancy and seeks to get a clean margin, which essentially is a certain border of clean tissue surrounding the tumor. If the margins are not clean, the surgeon will go back in at a later time and continue to cut around the area until they get enough healthy tissue to feel confident that they have removed the cancerous threat to the area. The upside to lumpectomies include the fact that they are less invasive procedures; women heal more quickly from lumpectomies; you will likely retain sensation in the breast, and they are often less emotionally traumatic that mastectomies as they often preserve the breast. The downside is that depending on how your doctor does getting clean margins, you may be in for multiple procedures. Just brace yourself for that. You shouldn't automatically expect lumpectomies to be a "one and done" type of scenario. But as you will learn as you go through this process, no matter what you opt, you will always encounter emotional highs and lows along this journey. I'll go into that more later, especially as it applies to life after treatment.

As mentioned, lumpectomies are much easier to recover from than mastectomies. Often times, with the exception of the scar, there is not much noticeable change to the affected breast. However, that all depends on the size and location of the tumor. Sometimes, the surgery and subsequent radiation can leave the breast looking less full than it did before or dented. There are some options for reconstruction depending on the size of the lump that is removed. There are partial implants, or procedures using your own body tissue from other parts to fill the gap. Of course, as with anything, the options are expanding every day. Sometimes, when one breast is affected and the other is clean, women may consider having a reduction done on the unaffected breast to help align both of them to a similar shape and size.

If a woman decides to go the mastectomy route, there are several types of surgeries currently available, any of which can be done on one breast or two depending on the situation. The basic concept of a mastectomy is to remove all of the breast tissue to remove the malignancies. The way I was able to explain it to people who were curious would be to think of an orange. If you peeled the orange, and took out the pulpy inside, and then put the skin back together, that's fundamentally what a mastectomy is like.

There are several types of surgeries that qualify as a mastectomy. There is a simple mastectomy which basically removes all of the breast tissue but leaves the lymph nodes (with the exception of the sentinel node) in place. Many times, this is the option for women who opt to do this as a prophylactic procedure. Then there is a modified, radical mastectomy. It removes the breast tissues and multiple lymph nodes, but does not touch the pectoral muscles. The radical mastectomy does the same as the modified, but also includes the muscles behind the breast. This typically is only done when the cancer has breached the chest wall or the muscles. A skin-sparing mastectomy removes the breast tissue through a smaller incision, and leaves the vast majority of the outer portion of the breast in place. This is done to facilitate reconstructive options. A nipple sparing mastectomy removes the interior breast tissue bit leaves the nipple and areola in place. (Yes, that means you likely will lose the nipple with the other options. Welcome to the Barbie boobs club!)

The pros for opting for a mastectomy include the following: little need for concern regarding clean margins, reduced risk of repeat surgical procedures and the emotional roller coaster that comes with that; lack of sensation means somewhat less pain (although for some women, this might also be a downside when it comes to intimacy); the emotional upside that comes with treating the disease in a very aggressive nature; a greater selection of reconstructive options. Also, a mastectomy might reduce the need for other treatments such as chemo or radiation depending on the individual situation, but this is very uniquely determined from one patient to the next.

There are so many options for reconstruction. Immediate reconstruction versus delayed reconstruction. With implants or using your own tissue (this can come from the stomach, back or butt). Sometimes reconstruction isn't an option or isn't preferred.

Some women use prosthetics. This always makes me think of one of survivor who is dear to my heart. She called me after learning I was diagnosed and was a source of great comfort and laughter. She informed me all about the benefits of prosthetics. She told me that in the heat of summer, you can keep them in fridge during the heat of summer as a quick cooling option. She also told me that if my husband was feeling frisky and I was not in the mood, I could give him that to play with and go take a nap. Talk about a win-win! She also warned me not to leave my boobs in my purse. Apparently her young grandson found hers one day and followed with some questions she didn't want to answer.

As for mastectomy-related reconstruction, if you are going to have radiation, there are additional factors to Radiation can cause tissue to shrink or shrivel. That effect is even more pronounced with implants. Given that, if you choose to go the implant route, then you will likely need to have temporary tissue expanders put in first, then go through radiation, before you can have your permanent implants. Otherwise, you might end up with shrinky dinks for boobs. As you might imagine, radiation can seriously warp the synthetic girls!

Let me fill you in a little bit on the tissue expander process. Essentially, they are put in place during the same surgery as a mastectomy. They are small sacs that your surgeon will gradually fill with saline. My husband wanted to know if he could be in charge of that process. He was hoping there was a button to press. In his mind, he was envisioning something like the old pump sneakers. Hey, like I said, maintaining your sense of humor is critical, and we did get a few chuckles at the expense of the expanders. Their purpose is to gradually stretch the pectoral muscles, the skin and remaining tissue to make room for the permanent implants. You will experience some pain after each fill, but nothing crazy. You should know that the expanders are very hard. They are by necessity. They need to be hard in order to create the inside-out pressure to stretch the muscles. As a result, they are not the most comfortable things in the world. They reminded me of bocce balls. Clearly, not the most fun for rolling over in the middle of the night.

The good news is that they are temporary. They eventually get exchange for your regular implants. There are currently two main considerations when choosing implants: Silicone or saline. There are of course pros and cons of each. There is the stigma with the silicone implants that makes you wonder about the risks if they rupture. According my research, the current thinking is that the blood stream does not absorb the silicone post-rupture. It hangs out in the cavity where the implant sits. But remember, I am no doctor. I am just sharing with you my understanding of these types of implants. Silicone implants tend to be softer and more natural looking than saline. Some people feel safer with the saline implants because in the case of rupture, the body just absorbs the saline (i.e. salt water). No big deal or worries from that perspective. The downside is, they feel slightly less natural and can have ripples in the implant which might look a little funny. Oh, and if they rupture, saline implants can flatten quickly. So I hate to admit it, but I picture a balloon flying around while air blows out of a pin hole before it flattens out like a big dud. Either way, regardless of which option you choose, they are equally more comfortable than the tissue expanders.

The exchange surgery will take place several months after you finish active treatment. Your body needs more time to heal especially from the radiation. My surgery was 8 months after I finished treatment. The recovery from the implant exchange surgery is much quicker and easier than the mastectomy/expander surgery. They usually go right in from the original incision, pop the expanders out and put in the new, fabulous girls. They sew you back up, and send you on your merry way that same afternoon. The only important thing to remember is to make sure that you follow your doctor's instructions regarding lifting, exercise, etc. These are your permanent babies. You want them to stay exactly where your doctor put them, and you want to be sure they heal well so you can feel as beautiful as you really are. No one wants their boobs to slide into their armpits… And yes, that can happen!

The other option for reconstruction is much newer, and pretty cool. In one of the "flap" procedures, the surgeon essentially uses your own body tissue to recreate your new breasts. Surgeons now can take tissue from the stomach, butt, thigh or back and transplant it. The tram flap and the Diep flap both take from your abdomen, whereas the latissimus dorsi flap takes from the upper back. The gluteal flap comes from your butt and the tug flap from your thigh. Ahh, such options to choose from! The upside is that the "material" used to make the breast is all natural and feels more like your old breasts than an implant. And of course, the obvious fact that if they are taking if from somewhere in your body, it's going to reduce the size of that body part. Woohoo, a two-for-one special! The downside is that it is a much harder surgery to recover from than implants because it involves more body parts, and muscles. Think about the abdomen and back, and how much you rely on those core muscles. A lot! Your lifestyle might very heavily weigh in on your decision. For me, having a 2 year old at the time, I just wanted to heal as quickly as possible, so while the idea of the flap was pretty cool, it didn't seem practical for me.

Another issue with reconstruction is the nipples. As I mentioned earlier, most mastectomy options tend to mean the loss of the nipple. This was a definitely weird concept for me. However, there is an upside. You don't have to worry about the old "high beams" when it's cold anymore. This was a nice unexpected perk for me. I was always self-conscious about this. But the downside is, you end up missing a body part. That's never a good feeling. There are several options for this. They can recreate a nipple from other body parts (similar in concept to the flap procedures as listed above, but obviously on a lesser scale). They can tattoo nipples on. I have seen some that were pretty decent looking. Or you can do nothing! Some women choose to do alternative tattoos, turning their new breasts into a beautiful work of art.

I remember having a very surreal conversation with my mother and my husband about this. I was saying how I was considering the "do nothing" option, and they suggested going with temporary tattoos. That snowballed into the suggestion of having "seasonal" nipples. Stars for July 4th, pumpkins for Halloween, Easter eggs, Christmas trees, turkeys. You might imagine the laughter that surrounded that conversation. My husband is always particularly amused when he can get my typically demure, polite mother to discuss something outrageous! She was the one suggesting the seasonal idea. What? This fell into that category of mine which I have affectionately dubbed "am I really discussing this with my family?"

There is also a longer term side effect from surgery that you should be aware of called lymphedema. This occurs in cases where the doctors need to take out lymph nodes during the surgery to test them for cancer cells. The more they take out, the higher the risk of lymphedema. Essentially, the lymph nodes are part of the lymphatic system. I personally am not an expert, but I will do my best to describe the lymphatic system as I understand it. Its primary function is to move fluid throughout the body and to support the immune and circulatory systems. When someone has cancer that is on the move, the first place it spreads beyond the breast area is the lymph nodes. In order to stage breast cancer, doctors will have to determine if there are tumor cells in the lymph nodes in the armpit area, and how many nodes are impacted. They will typically do a sentinel node biopsy during your surgery, and may potentially take more than the sentinel node if cancer is detected.

Once those nodes are gone, the rest of the body needs to pick up the slack. Sometimes, it's just not possible for the body to keep up, and the affected arms can collect fluid and swell. This can go all the way up to the hand and can be quite uncomfortable, and certainly upsetting as well. There are several things you can do to mitigate this condition. Your doctor will likely give you specific instructions on how to prevent flare ups. For example, they may advise you whether or not it is ok to use those arms to have blood drawn, or to have your blood pressure checked. It's also prudent to use gloves for house work and for gardening. Any injury to the skin can cause fluid to accumulate. Also, even though airplane cabins are pressurized, long flights can also trigger a flare up. Even vigorous exercise that involves the arms or dancing can contribute, especially if they occur in a hot location. Seriously, this new life is such a pain in the butt, isn't it? All these strange new things to learn about your body. Crazy!

Speaking of hot locations, I'm sorry to tell you that sitting in a sauna or a hot tub are pretty much a thing of the past for us girls. Excessive heat can definitely contribute to a lymphedema flare up. (Here's the one upside if cancer throws you into menopause. You will have your own personal sauna in the form of hot flashes! How exciting. Note the sarcasm…) There are certain stretches and exercises that can help prevent and manage the condition. You also may be eligible to have a lymphedema sleeve made for you. Those are designed to keep constant pressure on the affected arm and to keep the swelling to a minimum. There are even some physical therapists who specialize in lymphedema management. Who knew! It's important to check with your insurance for any possible coverage that might be available. Some will help with offsetting the costs. You might be surprised at different offerings available to you. You won't know unless you ask. Trust me, the insurance company isn't going to be nice enough to come forward and provide you with a list of all the things they will do for you. They are not that nice.

6. MANAGING A MASTECTOMY

My expertise in the subject of surgery is limited to my own personal experience. I learned so much during the process that I wish I had known up front. As such, I decided that managing a mastectomy warranted its very own chapter to help the sisters who go that route.

I chose the aggressive surgical approach because of the nature of my cancer, and my desire to be aggressive back. I knew that the diffused malignancies on the left side would require a mastectomy to that breast. I also had a lump in the right breast, and could have opted for the lumpectomy in that breast. Think of the difference between a diffused and a well-defined tumor as the difference between a fresh batch of fluffy snow and a nicely packed snow ball. As mentioned earlier, if you have cancer removed via a lumpectomy, getting clean margins (that nice wide section of healthy tissue surrounding the tumor) is essential. When tumors are diffused, you can't really get those margins because the cancer is scattered all over. The best option for getting it all out was a mastectomy. Since I had to do the mastectomy on the one, bilateral just made sense to me. I decided to get it over with and do them both at once. I felt that in my situation there was too much risk otherwise. Plus, I wanted to have a nice matching set of new girls when I was done.

I elected to have the bilateral modified radical mastectomy on the left and a skin sparing mastectomy on the right. I also had a lymph node dissection with the tissue expanders put in place to prepare for future implants. Having radiation in my treatment plan didn't allow for the permanent implants to be done up front. As I mentioned earlier, the radiation could cause the implants to shrink and pucker. No one wants that as a permanent new look.

Truth be told, waking up from surgery with the partially filled expanders in place did help ease the stress of losing both breasts. I remember looking down when I woke up and in my haze, looking down and thinking "hmm, that's not too terrible. They are actually kind of cute". Having been rather endowed in the boob region since I was 12, I have to admit, it was kind of nice to downsize. My back was happy as was my inner teenager who suffered so carrying those suckers around feeling out of place for years!

The surgery took about 7 hours in total. It went quickly for me because the meds were delightful. They gave me an anti-anxiety drug before I even left the waiting room. Rumor has it that I argued with them when they tried to put my surgical cap on. A friend of mine who was a nurse had gotten me a pink ribbon surgical cap, and I wasn't going into surgery without that fanciness on my head. Needless to say, I have zero recollection of this happening. I'd say my family suffered through the actual surgery more than I did.

Women have different emotional reactions to the whole concept of a mastectomy. It's important to note that every one of these emotions is completely legitimate and appropriate. Often times, women find themselves in a tangled web of several of these feelings. They manifest differently from one person to the next.

Some women truly mourn the loss of their breast. Some get angry at their breasts. Some struggle with their feminity afterwards. Some are unaffected emotionally, and move forward without them and never look back. Personally, I didn't react emotionally to the surgery or its implications at first. I was just resolute to do it and move forward. I had a sort of tunnel vision and was charging forward without much thought about anything other than getting through it. As much as I hate looking in the mirror and seeing scars, and do sometimes struggle to adjust to a new body shape, I viewed it this way. It was my breasts that brought the stigma of cancer into my life. They brought a fear and trauma into my world. Given that, I came to resent them, and wanted them gone. I was angry at this part of my body for betraying me and bringing this unwelcome intruder into my world.

An important concept for me to embrace was that the mastectomy didn't change who I was inside. I remember going into surgery expecting that I would wake up feeling different somehow, but truth be told, even as I was still in the haze of anesthesia, I felt like myself, just really sore. It didn't make me any less of a woman, any different of a person or any less special. I learned that being a woman was more than the sum of certain body parts, it's how I defined myself as a person. It was who I was at my core, in my heart and soul that mattered. I came to realize that did not change as a result of my surgery. It makes me think of the song lyric "they cut into my skin, and they cut into my body, but they will never get a piece of my soul." I can attest that is 100% true.

There really are two components to recovering from a mastectomy. There is the emotional side, and then there is the plain old physical recovery part. A mastectomy is a pretty major surgery. Although, before I had mine, several women who had been through it told me it's not as painful as you might expect. I remember thinking they must be lying. I remember fearing that I would feel every inch of that incision. In my mind, they were amputating two body parts and expected it to be excruciating. However, now that I have been through it, I completely agree with those women. Much of your nerve endings are removed with the breast tissue, so often times, there is very little pain at the incision site. Of course the funky flip side to that is there is usually very little sensation left at all, i.e. numb boobs! Some women have a really hard time with the loss of sensation.

What I experienced is more like a muscular pain. For me, it felt as though I had done a thousand push-ups rather than undergone a knife. It felt more like my muscles were battered and sore. The very first week, I was not strong enough to cut up my dinner. Talk about a feeble feeling. I was 34 years old and had to have my mom cut up my chicken for me. LAME! But every day I got a little bit stronger and eventually, over time, got back to normal. It's important to follow whatever physical therapy routine your doctor gives you to gain your range of motion. If you do not do what they say, it will become increasingly harder to move. The longer you wait to begin your exercises or stretches, the harder it will become.

As far as the surgery itself, be prepared, you will not likely be in the hospital very long post-surgery. The doctors want to get you out of there as quickly as possible to reduce the risk of infection. Hospitals have germs. There is no amount of bleach that can change that fact. I went home in less than 24 hours of coming out of anesthesia. That was daunting. Truth be told though, it is very difficult to get rest in the hospital. It's noisy and intrusive. Being home is a much more comfortable way to recover. (well, that is, unless you have noisy and intrusive relatives.)

For your ride home, it's very helpful to have extra pillows to prop your arms and to support your body. In fact, investing is extra pillows is definitely a smart idea going into surgery. You will get a lot of use out of them throughout your recovery. I also used one to brace the surgical site from the seat belt. That ride will likely not be the most fun you have had in a vehicle. Every bump and pothole made me cringe. And I lived an hour and a half from where I had my surgery. While I was grateful for the excellent care I received at the hospital, I was not thrilled with the travel involved. Unfortunately, I was not medicated enough to be knocked out for the ride home, and morphine makes me nauseous. Ok, so I admit, I am no fun to be around post-surgery.

When you get home, laying down and getting back out of bed will be a challenge for a while. This is mainly because you will be sore and your muscles will be weak. There are several options in managing this. You could do the old slow roll maneuver to get in and out of bed, but you won't have much strength in your arms to push yourself up. Sleeping in a recliner might be one of the best ways to get rest if it is an option for you. This is a great way to wrestle the lazy boy away from any man in your life. They can't deny you the comfy chair, you have cancer dammit! If you have jp drains in (which I will cover more in depth below), you want to be careful not to roll on them when you sleep. The results can be as gross as you might imagine. If you do lay down, consider propping yourself with as many pillows as possible. You might want them under your arms, your back, your neck and propped at your side to help secure you. I didn't sleep laying down until my drains actually came out.

One of the least pleasant parts of the whole post-surgical experience is the jp drains. They play an important role in healing, but let's call a spade a spade, they are as gross and uncomfortable as they sound! When the doctors told me about them, I dreaded them almost as much as I dreaded the overall surgery. They basically drain fluid out from the surgical site and look like plastic hand grenades at the end of long plastic tubes. It is kind of appropriate when you think about, who carries around hand grenades? Soldiers! So it makes sense that part of the battle against breast cancer arms us with hand grenades, no? That thought was one of the only ways I could amuse myself about that situation because aside from that, there is nothing fun about drains. I will say this, if you threw a full one of these suckers at an enemy, they would likely run the other way! So nasty.

The tubes are attached inside your body with a stitch (like I said, disgusting!). Because your body is adjusting to having a lot less tissue that was there before and may be missing some of the lymph nodes, excess fluid that would normally circulate through that area has nowhere to go. The drains help suction out the excess fluid, and it collects in the bulb. You will have to empty the drains several times a day in the beginning. That will decrease over time. Your doctor will ask you to monitor how much fluid drains daily, and use that as the indicator as to when they are ready to be removed.

Drains are everything you would anticipate. They add bulk under your clothes, which is not helpful as you might be struggling with body image to begin with. They can be slightly painful at the site where they are stitched in. Although if you find that they are extremely painful and if the area around it is inflamed, or if the gross stuff going into your drains smells funky, you might have an infection brewing. Keep in contact with your doctor if that happens. They are generally annoying and if you are not one for blood and guts, they are just plain yucky.

However, there are a few things you can do to help manage your drains, and make yourself a bit more comfortable. The tubing can be long and if not somehow secured, it can potentially be longer than your shirt. Let's be realistic, as much as your support group loves you, no one wants to see that nastiness! You can pin them to the inside of your shirt or to your bra. If you are crafty, you can make drain pouches that can fasten or velcro to your clothing. There are also some companies that make special tank tops or bras that have such pouches that attach to the garments or loops to which you can hook the drains. Google it!

Showering with drains can be particularly challenging. The very first shower I took, my cousin and I came up with a "brilliant" idea to wrap medical tape around my entire torso to secure the drains to my body. Sometimes, I swear the pain meds affected my judgment in the early days. While it was a comical sight, it was clearly not the most practical approach. Trust me, the last thing you need to do is to add to your list of challenges "peeling medical tape off of your entire body". We later learned that using a lanyard was a much easier way to keep the drains secured while trying to shower. I hooked the loops of the drains to a lanyard, tightened up and put it over my shoulder and viola! Much easier. Also, I recommend getting a shower chair, and a hand held shower head for the early post-surgery showers. You will find both to be helpful. You will have difficulty washing your own hair for a while, so these two objects might make it easier for whomever is assisting you. Don't be too discouraged if the act of showering exhausts you in the early days. I took a two hour nap after my first one!

Also, you will have a surgical bra to wear after you come home, which is basically a more sterile looking version of a sports bra. Because your body can swell, the bra can dig into your skin. One way to help relieve this is to tuck a gauze pad under the edge of the bra. This will provide a buffer and will make it much more comfortable. Sadly, it took me about 2 weeks to figure that one out. When I had my implant exchange, I was happy to have learned from my previous experience.

Your recovery from surgery will take time. Allow yourself to heal. Finding the balance between being active enough, and not overdoing it can be a challenge. Do what you can to make yourself as comfortable as possible. Clothing is an important component of that. Zip-up shirts with pockets in the front were my uniform as I healed from surgery. It will be a while before you can lift any shirts over your head, so having a zip-up or button up option is key. The pockets helped because I found myself bowing my arms out around the drains and the swelling in the early days, which made my arms very tired. Having the pockets allowed me to rest my arms when I needed too while keeping them away from my body.

Also, in the beginning, you will likely want to prop your arms with pillows no matter what you are doing. It helps promote drainage and it makes things a bit more comfortable. I propped everywhere, on the couch, in the chair, even at the kitchen table. Make yourself as comfortable as you can when you rest. The rest is so critical to healing. You will be more tired than usual in the days and weeks following the surgery. Remember, that your body is generating scar tissue and doing some major healing. It takes time and energy to do that. Don't expect to go about your normal business. It's just not practical.

Do yourself a favor. Ask your doctor and your insurance company about a visiting nurse service. Often times, for this type of surgery, insurance plans will allow for this because while they prefer to get you home from the hospital quickly, you really still do require care. The nurses will be quite helpful in making sure you are ok and providing you with personal attention and answer any questions you may have along the way. Their presence will be quite comforting in those early days in your new body. Let them take good care of you. That's what they are there for.

I have a funny story to share about my first visiting nurse experience. The day after I returned home from my surgery, the nurse came to check on me. Up until that point, my mom and my cousin had been my primary caretakers, and they watched me like a hawk, while my husband tended to our son. Part of the nurse's routine was to examine the incision sites and ensure everything looked like it was healing well. So we marched into the bathroom, followed by my cousin and my mother. What happened next was a combination of surreal and comical. The nurse removed the bandages and instantly commented on how everything looked great. My cousin and mom were both pleasantly surprised as well, and had no problem saying so. Talk about bizarre! I felt like a marble statue in a museum being stared at. Mind you, prior to my surgery, I was incredibly modest, and never even wore anything too revealing. Here I was, standing in the middle of the room, half naked, with my surgically altered breasts hanging out, with an audience admiring my new "girls". Yikes! And when my mom blurted out "Oh you will be so happy", well, that took the cake. We all couldn't help but laugh. Um, thanks Mom. I think. Not exactly something I ever expected to hear immediately following a double mastectomy. But at least they didn't gasp in horror. I guess we can be grateful for small favors.

While they were able to gawk unabashed at my new breasts, admittedly, it took me quite a while to be able to even peak at them myself. Each patient should only do that when they are ready. It is a change, and it can be very traumatic. So take your time, and go easy on yourself. It took me a couple of weeks to really comfortably look at my incisions. At first, I started by just using peripheral vision, then I moved to glancing at the reflection in the glass shower door. It took a while before I was able to look at them directly in the mirror. Once I did, I gradually grew more comfortable with them. Before I had the tissue expanders filled, I remember thinking that they looked like little, pathetic atrophied boobs compared to what I was used to. Sad, sweet little shriveled things. The surgeon had left enough extra skin to accommodate the eventual expansion and reconstruction, and at that time, had not been filled out. As much as I thought they had a pathetic way about them, I didn't mind. They were healthy and that was what mattered. As the filling process went on, they got that perkiness that I never quite experienced before. In the end, I found that they turned out quite alright. I'm looking forward to be in the Senior Citizens' development one day where I will surely be the envy of the other old bitties who are slaves to the over-the-shoulder boulder holders! Take that suckas!

One of my scars actually makes me smile. Due to the location of the tumor, they couldn't cut it straight across. The resulting scar looks very much like the hill and valley of a roller coaster. I noticed that the very first time that I saw it, and I smiled at the beautiful irony of it as the whole cancer experience was certainly the most wild ride I have ever ridden. I even considered having the scar turned into a tattoo of a roller coaster, but I wimped out. The whole physical change was an adjustment, but in time, I learned to embrace my battle scars, and I now look at them with pride of all that I have accomplished. They are a sign of strength for me.

You will get to know your new body under your own terms. Remember this, your breasts probably only account for at most 10% of your body (and I am sure my numbers are not quite right but you get the point I am about to make). That means that even if you have a double mastectomy, 90% of your body is not impacted by this disease. Learn to still love yourself. Yes, you may be different, but you are still beautiful. You are strong and resilient, and you have the scars to prove it. Be proud of your body and all it can endure. And remember, your physical appearance is just the outer shell for your soul. That is the core of you. That is the part that really matters. That is what will leave a mark on this world. Not your body or what any part of it looks like.

Recovering from surgery takes time and patience. You need to find the fine balance between pushing yourself and knowing your limits so you don't jeopardize your healing. Your body will not likely let you do too much, especially in the early days. Your body is generating tissue, building scars and recovering. It was just through something incredibly traumatic. I remember being so mad that I was so exhausted after my first shower that I needed to take a nap. I felt pathetic, but it was very normal. Learn to listen to your body. It knows best what it needs to heal. It knows better than you do. Trust me on this one.

You also should talk to your doctor about physical activity. The sooner you are able to start light exercise, the better. It helps promote blood flow which is always good for healing. It also helps stretch out the muscles which improves mobility. It will improve your general health. Don't expect to be able to run a 5k the week after surgery, but you should be able to gradually increase your exercise, and each time you do, you will feel increasingly better.

7. CHEMO!

Ah, yes. Chemo! Indeed, it's a beast, but for many a breast cancer sister, chemotherapy is a critical part of treatment. As much as no one ever wants to do it, sometimes, it's often the best insurance for a longer, healthier, happier life. I do believe the phrase "necessary evil" might have been coined with chemo in mind.

Chemotherapy is essentially chemical warfare on cancer. It can come in different forms, but the two main ones are intravenous or pill. The point of chemo is to kill any random cancer cells that are floating around in your body, or to reduce any cancer that is unable to be treated in other ways. If you have cancer in your lymph nodes, likelihood is, your medical oncologist is going to recommend some form of chemo. The reason for this is that once it hits that lymphatic system, it's flowing around your body, and if it feels feisty enough, it could grab hold somewhere and metastasize. The mission of chemo is to hunt down those little suckers and poison them in their tracks. Think of a pest control service bombing a house that has termites. Chemo gets cancer in places where it might not be obvious. Unfortunately, the side effects pop up because chemo affects healthy cells as well. That's the bummer.

There are so many different types of chemotherapy drugs available and each one has a unique list of effects on the body. Even if you do not have the same chemo regimen as I did, the focus is on managing the side effects which you may encounter regardless of the specific drugs involved. Many drugs have several similar effects on the body. First things first, you will likely have to determine your chemo side effects pattern. Typically, from one cycle to the next, you will see a trend emerging as the drugs work their way through your system. I would suggest that you get a little pocket calendar and track each day what side effects you have. You generally will see the pattern emerge through each cycle, and then as time goes on, you will be able to better manage the side effects once you know what to expect as your normal. By the end of your second cycle, if you watch closely, and work with your medical team, you should be able manage them pretty well.

Before you start chemo, be sure that you are comfortable with your oncologist and their support staff. It is so critical that you feel at ease going to them with questions, and speaking honestly with them. You are likely to have conversations about topics that you never expected to discuss in your lifetime, and these topics are probably pretty awkward for you. Don't forget though, they are normal for your doctor. This is what they see every day, so don't be embarrassed to ask any questions, not matter what the topic or bodily function is involved.

You also want to be sure that you feel that you are a priority to them. You need them to be responsive. Make sure you know how to get in touch with them at any given time because you do not know when a chemo issue will crop up. I am willing to bet you that at some point during your experience, something will come up at an odd time that you will need to discuss with them and it will not be able to wait until your next appointment.

Expect that you will be in contact with them between visits, and do not be afraid to reach out to them.

Some practitioners become apathetic about oncology patients because that is all they see, so they become desensitized. In their world, a cancer patient is just like everyone else they see. Some practitioners forget: being a chemo patient is a big deal! Make sure they treat you as such. Hopefully, this is the first (and only) time you are going through this, so it is natural that you might have a lot of questions. Your body is going through a lot of intense stuff that is likely all new to you. As such, you need to have unfettered access to your medical team. Side effects will happen. Expect them. They are not fun, but they are usually controllable. It will take communicating openly and regularly with your team to know exactly what you can do to minimize them. The solutions are not usually intuitive to what you typical might do in the real world, so you will need to rely on the experts to guide you. You will get through it. Just be patient and take it one day at a time.

As prep for your treatment, you might be given the option for a chemo port. Some doctors believe in them, and some don't. Essentially, a port is a little disc-shaped object that gets placed in your chest or arm. Chemo drugs can sometimes cause your problems with your veins that make it difficult to get stuck so often, so a port helps mitigate that issue. It basically hooks up to your vein, and helps the drug go straight into your blood stream. Depending on the size of the port, you will probably be able to see it. It looks like a little bruised lump. Lovely! Nosey people will probably ask you what it is. I was lucky, I don't know why, but the doc who put mine in opted to go with a pediatric sized one, so that was a bit less noticeable. He said it had something to do with my tissue expanders.

Ports have their pros and cons, like anything else in life, of course. They do make getting stuck every time you go for treatment a bit easier because you don't have to worry about your doc finding a vein each time. They just pop in the needle and you are done 1-2-3. The downside is that like any foreign object, it's an infection risk. When you have a chemo port, any time you get a fever (which is possible to happen during chemo, especially if you have the immune boosting drugs) you need to go to the ER. They need to check to see if your port is infected, and to see if your immune system is strong enough to fight it off. The nice part about it was that they tend to get you a private room if one is available because your immune system is compromised. That is a nice perk.

I had 5 ER runs during my time in chemo. The first time it happened, I cried my eyes out. Everything out of the ordinary scared me, and of course the very thought of going to the ER scared me. After a while though, it got a little less scary. The last trip happened to be on our 7th wedding anniversary. Poor Steve, he was living up to the "in sickness and in health" part of the vows that night. So our romantic celebration consisted of a stop at the drive thru on the way to the hospital, and watching Harry Potter between blood work and chest x-rays. Good times!

Ports also need to be flushed regularly to prevent infection and clotting. And the sooner you can get that sucker out, the better. I have a cousin who still has hers in from her cancer fight over 5 years ago. Hey, Cugina! If you are reading this, you know who you are. Get it out! Get going!

So, what can you expect on treatment day? It's really not so bad. They usually have comfy recliners for the patients in the infusion suite. I always bought a bag of entertainment with me. I had time to kill, so I brought a laptop, some crocheting, books, music, a few snacks and a chemo buddy. You can't go anywhere for a few hours, so you need to find ways to amuse yourself. Usually, your day will start with blood work. They need to make sure your chemo hasn't crapped out your blood cells or immune system before they load you up with more poison. Once they get clearance, they call down for the pharmacy to mix up your fancy chemo cocktail. Then once that arrives, it's game time. They stick you like a pin cushion, and start the pre-meds. This is often consists of steroids, antacids and anti-histamines. The point of them is to basically help your body cope with the meds. Then they start the big drip. You have nothing to do but to sit and let the chemo do its job of flowing into your veins. So you have a few hours to veg. It's actually kind of weird, but nice to have down time. There is nowhere to go, and nothing really to do but relax. Once you hear the lovely beep of the machine, you know your treatment is done, and you go on your merry way and wait for the side effects to start.

And trust me, in due time, they will come…

So, let's talk side effects, shall we? When most people hear the word chemo, it conjures up images of bald people bowing to the porcelain god. Nausea is the one side effect that has become synonymous with chemo. Come on, let's face it. There is no one in this world who likes puking, or who could even remotely truthfully say "eh, barfing doesn't bother me much". Bull! It sucks! Luckily, medical technology has advanced the management of this side effect from what it was years ago. Most patients are able to get some relief from this dreaded affect. There are several drugs available that help quell it. Do not be afraid to take them according to the prescription. There's no trophy for making it through chemo without taking nausea meds. The very first night following my initial infusion, I set my alarm clock to the time when I was due to take my next dose. My nausea woke me up 5 minutes before the alarm went off! I kid you not. I was shocked at how precise the timing was. From that point on, I took the drugs exactly as scheduled, and was very lucky! I never threw up during chemo. There is no need to suffer unnecessarily, nor to risk dehydration when there are options to help manage the side effect. Rather, be grateful to modern science for the wonders of the anti-nausea meds.

Tandem to the nausea is food aversions and cravings. Chemo can affect the way things taste and smell. I don't know why this is, but it's very true. It screws up your taste buds something fierce. Foods taste completely different than they did pre-chemo. Similarly, many women report a heightened sense of smell where you seem to notice every little scent. I couldn't stand the smell of coffee when I was going through treatment. It literally made me gag. This was particular rough for someone who drank a minimum of two cups a day prior to cancer. Also, many people get a funny taste in their mouths that just won't go away. For me, it was a very sour taste. For my mom, it was a super sweet taste, another survivor said she tasted metal. Whatever changes occur to your taste buds ultimately affect the way foods then taste. There really are a lot of similarities to chemo and pregnancy. I marveled at this. One of my favorite people on the planet was pregnant while I was going through chemo. We often compared notes because our symptoms overlapped. She was getting ready to give birth to a beautiful baby boy, and I was getting ready to be reborn myself. An interesting parallel, no doubt.

You very well might find some of your favorite foods are no longer appealing while you are going through chemo. I remember a story of a dear family friend who was going through treatment and really wanted a glass of wine to relax. She took a sip of one and thought that bottle had gone bad. She opened a different one, and that too tasted awful. By the third opened bottle, she realized that it was because of the changes in her taste buds. She was livid!

You also might find that you crave certain foods. For me, I craved macaroni and cheese and pork fried rice. Not the healthiest of choices by any stretch, but it helped soothe the queasiness and for whatever reason, that's what my body wanted at the time. So I went with it. And yes, I gained 7 pounds during chemo. But I didn't fret it too much. I was grateful to get through it. Weight Watchers was waiting on the other side for me.

Another related side effect that some encounter is mouth sores. This obviously can also hinder your ability to eat. The lining of your mouth and throat may become raw as your body is unable to regenerate those cells. There are a few things that you can do to help. Avoid eating or drinking acidic food or beverages. As you might imagine, this can be horribly painful if you have an open sore. Also, use a baking soda based tooth paste and a soft bristle tooth brush just to be a little more gentle. They have peroxide-based mouth washes that are designed to help with sores. Definitely investigate this and keep it handy. If you find your pain gets unbearable, your doctor can likely prescribe you something called a "magic mouthwash" (yes, that's the real name) which is a combo of liquid meds that you swish around to numb the mouth and help ease the pain.

Hair Loss is other side effect that is typically ubiquitous with chemo. Not all chemo drugs and cancer patients lose their hair, but most breast cancer drugs do cause it. It tends to be more traumatic for several reasons. To me, it was the tell-tale sign that there was something wrong with me. I could walk around after my mastectomy, and no one would know what I had been through, but that wasn't the case with the hair loss. It was the sign to the rest of the world that told them I had cancer. It was my scarlet letter. In our culture, hair is part of the feminine mystique. Most of our lives, it's very much a part of our style. We are surrounded by images of gorgeous locks of hair in the media. Knowing that we are going to lose it is a pretty daunting prospect. What was amazing to me was that my oncology nurse was able to predict to the day when the majority of the hair would come out. In my case, it was day 17 after my first infusion.

Around day 10, I noticed my hair was starting to thin, so I embraced my inner GI Jane, and had my head buzzed. My cousin has been a barber for 30 years, and agreed to come to the house to do it. We both were nervous and didn't know how we would handle the moment when it happened, but I was resolute. It helped me to take matters into my own hands. It was pretty wild to see all of my hair on the floor when it was over. It was pretty intense. I realized how much I looked like my older brother. I also realized how dark my hair really was. Having colored my hair for the better part of 10 years, I had no clue what my natural color was anymore. It was pretty funny to realize that it was close to jet black (well, aside from the greys that were growing in). I also realized how empowering it was to control the terms of losing my hair. Granted, I was going to lose it due to chemo, but it made me feel a little bit more in charge. Plus it gave me time to gradually get used to the idea rather than waiting until the majority of it fell out in one fell swoop.

On the day it came out, I was at my parents' home. I remember my head felt weird. It's a hybrid of an itchy, tingly, mildly sore sensation. I got into the shower, and scrubbed my head until all of the lose pieces fell out. It took a long time, but my head felt so much better once it was. In the midst of the tears that were streaming down my face along with the shower water, I ended up chuckling. I realized halfway through the ordeal that I was using volumizing shampoo! I laughed loudly and thought to myself, "well, that's not going to live up to its claims today, is it?" I had the whim of sending them a picture with a complaint that their product made my hair fall out, but I decided I couldn't be that cruel.

There are a lot of options for head coverings. I lived in a thin ski cap for most of the time because it was the most comfortable for me. I did get two wigs for when I didn't feel like looking like a cancer patient. I had a gorgeous one I called my "fancy girl" that I wore to nice social occasions and work. I had a baseball cap with a wig sewn underneath that another survivor friend gave to me. I loved that one. It was my go-to in most daily outings. Some women wear scarves. I was never stylish enough to pull that look off. Others wear baseball caps. And some women are just awesome enough to rock the bald look. This can be just so beautiful, especially paired with pretty earrings. I think it screams in the face of cancer saying "screw you!" It's a bold, strong look. I never was confident enough to pull that off anywhere but around my home or occasionally in the car.

If you do get a wig, I highly recommend checking with your insurance carrier to see what coverage you might have available to you. Many insurance policies have a stipulation that allows some sort of reimbursement for wigs for cancer patients. There are a few things you should know. Call first to find out the rules of your plan. Write down the date of this discussion and exactly what they told you. When I was later appealing the denial of my claim, having this information was incredibly helpful. They likely will require that your oncologist write a prescription for a "cranial prosthesis". Yes, that is the medical insurance terminology for wig! I have to admit, that made me laugh. You will likely need to submit the paperwork after paying for the wig out of pocket. Then you need to prepare yourself for a fight. Several women I have known have had to argue with their insurance companies because they subsequently denied coverage. I am going to let you in on a little secret. Insurance companies are businesses. They want to hang onto as much money as they can, so sometimes they deny claims that they shouldn't deny in the hopes that you will give up and they get a bonus. Sad, but true. It took me a year to get my reimbursement check for my wig. They denied me for a few reasons. My favorite was when they told me they denied me because they didn't have my diagnosis code in the system. Listen dudes, it's 174.9. I cringe every time I see it on paperwork. But in that moment, I laughed and replied, "then what the hell did you approve the double mastectomy, chemo, radiation and tamoxifen for?" Needless to say, that help drive home the point. But I still had to fight with them for several more months before I got reimbursed. Truth be told, I fought cancer, I was sure as hell not going to allow some stupid insurance company stand in my way! Jerks, picking on the cancer patient!

You also might want to consider a program sponsored by the American Cancer Society called "look good, feel better." It's a wonderful program that helps women learn tips to help them manage the inevitable changes to their appearance. They talk about head coverings, and often give you make-up tips to help you feel better. American Cancer Society (bless their hearts) also has a great catalogue of head coverings that includes wigs, hats, and scarves at a very inexpensive price. I never made it to one of these sessions, but everyone I know who did absolutely loved it! Truth be told, just about any program run by ACS is going to be pretty awesome.

About a month after I lost my hair, I connected with a friend who was going through breast cancer treatment as well. She was a few weeks behind me in her journey. She told me she had heard of a treatment in Europe to prevent hair loss called "cold caps". It can be quite expensive, but by wearing the cap, the theory is, it freezes the hair follicles and reduces the amount of chemotherapy drugs that it can absorbed, therefore preserving the hair. From what she explained to me, it was pretty intense wearing the cap, but it did work for her. Her hair thinned slightly, but she never really lost it. If I had this information ahead of time, I am not sure what choice I would have made regarding this. It certainly is appealing to not have to go through the hair loss and regrowth process, but considering it is also painful, I don't know if I would have decided to go that route or not. It's an individual woman's choice: the emotional pain of the hair loss, or the physical pain to retain it. The other thing to consider is the fact that the scalp would not receive the chemotherapy, and while that is an area of the body that is extremely rarely affected by wandering cancer cells, it's a risk, albeit a very small one.

Here are some websites that speak to the cold caps in case you are interested.

- http://rapunzelproject.org/ColdCaps.aspx

- http://www.washingtonpost.com/wp-dyn/content/article/2011/01/10/AR2011011006036_2.html?tid=wp_ipad&sid=ST2011011702804

Tangent to the hair loss, some drugs can affect your finger nails and toe nails. The same concept that applies to the hair applies here. The rapidly growing cells that create healthy nails can get disrupted. This side effect though is often a longer term one that you won't notice right away. Basically, the nail beds can come loose because the cells that bind the nail to the skin are not keeping up to speed. You might find your nails become discolored or dented. You might find them weaker, or you might find them coming loose. The best thing you can do is keep your nails as short as possible. This will reduce your risk of inadvertently hitting them and popping them off before they are fully ready (and yes, it is as painful as you might think). If they do lift during treatment, remember that you are more prone to infection. Keep an eye on them, and if you notice anything funky, make sure you tell your doctor. You might need an antibiotic to help it heal. It can take a while before the process is fully over. At the time of this writing, I was 8 months post-treatment, and I lost another toenail just last week. Thankfully, a replacement grew in its place before it came off, so it didn't hurt and still looks pretty, which is good considering it was July and flip flop season was here!

Fatigue is another common side effect that most people encounter. The severity of it varies based on the drug and the dosage, but no matter what, expect that your energy levels will be affected. It's pretty much a given. The range could be anywhere on the spectrum from just needing to go to bed a little early all the way to having some days where you cannot get out of bed at all. You usually will notice a pattern and will be able to prepare yourself for the days that will be the worst. In my case, it was always Sundays. It became affectionately known in my world as "Chemo Sundays". I remember one particular Chemo Sunday when my friend and coworker came to visit. I had sent my son and husband out for the day. I spent most of the day drifting in and out of sleep while my friend kept me company. I stood up at one point to make some macaroni and cheese, and was too tired to stand up long enough to stir the pasta while it cooked. My friend had to do it for me. I just couldn't. It was very hard for me to accept that there would be days when I was really very useless for anything other than watching mindless tv. Although these became the days when I was grateful for bad reality shows. Somehow, I didn't feel so guilty wasting brain cells watching.

Interestingly enough, you would think with the fatigue, you would have no trouble sleeping while on chemo. Some days, this is absolutely true. Other days, the exact opposite is the case. Insomnia is a huge issue during cancer treatment, particularly during chemo. There are a few contributing factors to this. One big cause is the use of steroids during treatment. Many chemo drugs use meds like decadron to mitigate the side effects of the chemo drug. Unfortunately, this has its own side effect that tends to be particularly prevalent in the 48 hours following treatment: Sleeplessness. I cannot tell you how much writing, crocheting and just plain staring at the ceiling occurred at 3 am following the decadron. The bummer was, the rest of the world was sleeping and I was bored and pumped on steroidal energy! Not a good mix. The other cause of insomnia is the stress that comes with cancer. My mind was often in overdrive due to the fears, worries and concerns of my situation. I relied heavily on mediation to help distract my mind and relax. It was a concerted effort, no doubt. I am eternally grateful to the internet as there were plenty of guided meditations for me to listen to in order to manage this issue.

Going into treatment, I expected I would do a lot of reading. I always loved to read, but as an adult rarely found the time to carve out for it. I reveled the idea of days on end of having nothing to do but rest and read. To be honest, I couldn't focus long enough to comprehend anything I was reading, so it was pointless for me. What a huge bummer! Sometimes, I was just that tired. And truth be told, with chemo brain (which I address later) my reading comprehension was not so good. I was pretty pleased when treatment was over and my brain was less foggy and I could indulge in a good book again.

Some women also experience pain while going through treatment. The severity can vary. It could be bone pain (which can be exacerbated by the immune boosting drugs that are often prescribed during treatment), joint pain, or just general soreness. It can pop up in various parts of the body. Many women experience pain in the back and hips. I remember the most random pain I had was in the joint of my pinkie finger. Bizarre! The immune boosting drug for me was a mild ache, but for my mom was a severe pain. It can vary from individual to individual. When I was on Taxol, the pain in my joints was sharp. It felt like someone was stabbing my bones with a thousand sharp tooth picks. Bizarre and very uncomfortable.

Some aches and pains might be manageable with just using over the counter pain meds, while some experience pain that requires much more pain management. If it is debilitating enough, talk to your doctor about prescription pain meds to help you keep it to a manageable level. It's important to stay ahead of the pain. By that, I mean, don't wait for the pain medication to completely wear off before taking the next dose. Take them according to the schedule. So if it says take it every 4 hours, do so. Don't wait… Like I said about nausea, there is no medal for getting through it without meds. You are no less of a hero if you take something to manage side effects. And don't take it more frequently than you are told. That is never a good idea.

Taxol/Taxotere has a unique side effect called neuropathy. It basically is a chronic pins and needles or numb feeling in the hands or feet. It tends to come on gradually. It can range from annoying to debilitating. I remember reading once that Melissa Etheridge opted against the drug because she was concerned about neuropathy affecting her livelihood, i.e. her ability to play the guitar. Can't say I blame her. What a tough choice in her situation!

Digestive issues are the often unspoken side effects. They are uncomfortable and not pleasant to talk about, but if I am going to help someone, the only way to do so is to be honest so that they may know what to expect. So bear with me on this journey down Gross Road. Going into chemo, a friend of mine told me about how she suffered with some of these. I was surprised to hear it because these are some of the side effects that no one talks about because presumably, it's too taboo. Once in treatment, I was so very grateful to know that it was common or I might have panicked.

I'll start with an easy one: acid reflux/indigestion. Remember, chemo affects rapidly dividing cells. As such, most linings are susceptible to irritation. This includes your throat, esophagus, and your stomach. Acid can really cause an issue, when the linings are already sensitive and not regenerating as quickly as usual. Talk to your doctor about what you can to do get relief. You may be able to take antacid medication. You may have to adjust your diet. I found that my stomach couldn't handle acidic foods for about a week after chemo. This included foods such as tomato sauce, anything vinegar based, (both of which are devastating for an Italian-American like me), citrus fruits, etc. The pain from eating things like this when your insides are raw is pretty intense. I even had them put meds in my chemo bags to help ease the side effects.

Now for the more awkward, gross stuff: constipation vs. diarrhea. Yummy! While in the general course of life, what I am about to discuss falls into the realm of "TMI" (too much information, in the land of cancer, these are every day hurdles. I was eternally grateful to survivor who warned me of these because they would have freaked me out! These are topics no one ever wants to discuss, but in the name of honesty, here goes.

Many of the drugs can cause one of these two side effects. Unfortunately, there is no way to know which of the two you will get ahead of time, or to even know if you will get either of them. It's a wait and see game. Obviously, if you get "going too much" problem, there are several risks, you could end up stripping the good bacteria out of your intestines, and you run the risk of dehydration, and other complications such as c-diff. Managing this side effect can be important to stay strong so that you can continue with your treatment. Ask your doctor about medications to help manage this. Likelihood is that they will end up prescribing an anti-diarrheal medication and might also suggest the use of probiotics to help.

If you have the opposite problem, the constipation will be like no constipation you have ever known. I have been pregnant and dealt that version, trust me. This is different and worse! This is not your run-of-the mill constipation. This is more like having your insides shut down completely and turn into cement regardless of what you put into your body. If you think of it as a machine that processes the stuff that you put in your mouth, it literally feels like someone pulled the plug on the machine, and nothing moves.

For me, it literally felt like my intestines were being filled with concrete. And it felt like the surrounding walls were concrete as well. Moving anything through there (even with all the stool softeners in the world) seemingly took an act of God. Talk about uncomfortable, painful, and downright yucky! That literally was one of the worst of the chemo side effects for me. It literally kept me home bound, uncomfortable and in pain for the majority of the time. And being as it's so gross, I didn't tell most people about it. I just said I was "home managing side effects" and left it at that because really, who wants to hear about someone else's pooping problems? No one. Ever…

Sometimes, the medications that you take to manage the side effects can cause other side effects. Some of the anti-nausea meds can exacerbate the constipation issues. So it comes down to the lesser of the two evils. Do you want to puke your guts up or have every food item just go into lock down in your system?

Oh joy, what a choice! Ok, enough of that grossness. Whew. On to other side effects that are a little less gruesome...

There are a lot of factors that can delay treatment, many of which are well beyond your control. Some of which are a result of side effects. You will always have to have blood work the day of your treatment to determine if you are cleared to get chemo. The reason for this is that chemo can affect your red blood cells, iron count and white blood cells among other things. There is not much you can do to control this. Talk to your doctor each treatment to understand how your blood work looks and what you can do about it. Be aware that the changes in your counts could affect your immune system, so be extra vigilant about germs. Your body is working very hard to kick cancer, so it might be using up resources that you might normally use to ward off the common cold, etc. Be sure to be careful about exposure to germs. Wash your hands frequently. Communicate your status with people around you so they are mindful to steer clear of you if they are ill in any way. A small cold can become a much bigger deal to someone with a compromised immune system.

If you and your doctor feel it is ok for you to work part-time during chemo, and if you have the option to work remotely, please do so. I personally found working was a welcome distraction for me. But it wasn't worth the risk of going to an office with 100 other people during the height of cold and flu season. I realize that some people might not have the choice, but if it is available to you, please, please consider it. It's not worth the risk. You could end up hospitalized and that would only delay treatment. You just want to get this nonsense over as quickly as you can.

This last side-effect is truly one of my favorites. Yes, believe it or not, not all about chemo is terrible, if you keep your sense of humor. Let me start by saying this: chemo brain is real! Studies show it, and when you are living it, you realize it's no joke. It can be frustrating at times, but often times when you look back on it, you are able to laugh because it is so ridiculous. For example, when you confuse the preparation H for the toothpaste. Yes, that really happened. And, more importantly, yes, I realized it before it went in my mouth! YUCK!

I asked several survivors to share with me their chemo brain stories. My favorite response was the one dear survivor who told me "I don't remember". That, my friends is chemo brain. It's a fog that literally zaps your short term memory and ability to focus. Sometimes, you do things without realizing you are doing them. Often times, it makes details very fuzzy to recall. So enjoy the stories, and as you encounter them yourself, try to laugh them off. I personally enjoyed this side effect because I was a scatter brain before I had cancer, and now I had an awesome excuse to blame it on!

One morning, post-treatment, I was getting my son ready for school, and walked with him into the garage to my van. When I got there, I thought that I had left the keys in the car. Fortunately (or so I thought it was fortunate) I had left the window open. So I reached in, and unlocked the window. The alarm went blaring off. I didn't even know I had an alarm! So I scurry back into the house with my child and arms full of our lunch boxes, his backpack, my purse, and start running around like a nut looking for my keys. My son was standing there stunned with his hands over his ears, clearly stunned by what just happened. I ran around for a few minutes, with the blaring alarm heightening my stress. My keys were nowhere to be found. I walked back into where I had tossed the bags, and the keys were sitting there tossed with them. I had them in my hand the whole time.

Many a chemo brain mishaps seem to be kitchen-centric. For example, there was the time I cut up veggies to bring to work as a snack. When I got to my office, I reached into my lunch bag to indulge in my healthy treat, only to find it was missing. For the life of me, I couldn't figure out what I did with them. I thought maybe I put them in my son's lunchbox. When I got home from work, and was prepping dinner, I found the bag I had prepared hanging out in the veggie drawer. In my fog, I apparently put them back in the fridge when I was cleaning up on my way out the door. The good news was that they didn't go to waste. Then there was the time I went to put cinnamon in my oatmeal, only to realize it was paprika! That would have been nasty.

My mom's favorite chemo brain moment came in when she went to meet with the genetic counselor for the first time. The counselor asked her for her medical history. So she started recounting what she had been through to date. Then, when she went to describe her tumor profile, she told the counselor that she was BRCA Negative. The counselor looked at her kindly and said "how could you know that if this is the first time we are meeting? You haven't had your BRCA test yet". My mother laughed, and said "oh sorry, chemo brain! I meant the thing that you treat with herceptin. I forget what that is called." (i.e. the Her2 protein). At least she was able to laugh about it.

Fridge/freezer mix-ups seem to be a common occurrence. I remember spinning around in my kitchen going from one cabinet to the next while trying to cook dinner because I couldn't remember where I kept anything. I have several times put things in the freezer that did not belong there including boxes of cereal. A dear friend of mine reports putting salad in the freezer, which of course she didn't find until a few days later and by that point, the salad had to be tossed. She also reports having put paper towels on the bottom of the shopping cart, paying for them, but forgetting to put them in the truck, therefore losing them.

Things became extremely comical when I was through treatment and my mom was in the middle of hers. Our conversations were pretty pathetic because inevitably one of us would forget the details of the story we were trying to tell. It must have been pretty painful to listen to us. I think over the course of a year and a half, we probably never finished more than two conversations without getting distracted.

One of the most noticeable effects of chemo brain for me personally was it hampered my sense of time. I have a very difficult time keeping track of what day it is and what was scheduled for when. Now, those who know me might chuckle and say that was not a result of chemo brain, but trust me. It was grossly exacerbated by chemo. I completely forgot doctor's appointments not realizing what day it was.

Truth be told, sometimes chemo brain produces some pretty funny stories, but it also can be incredibly frustrating. Cognitive difficulties are somewhat unnerving and can be frustrating. It can be particularly challenging if you return to work after (or even during) treatment. I found for me, it was much harder to focus, concentrate and remember things. My short term memory was terrible following chemo. Admittedly, it made going back to work a tremendous challenge for me. I had to get organized and fast or I would never have accomplished anything. My ability to retain a thought, and remember to do something was severely compromised. Working was a lot more of a mental effort than it ever was before.

This is where modern technology, or old-fashioned organizational skills can come in handy. There are plenty of tools to help you keep track of your life. Use them! I have often had a random thought, and if I didn't write it down or plug it into my phone, it would have been lost forever. I rely heavily on reminders in my phone to keep me on track. If I think of something I need to do in the morning, I will never remember to do it in the afternoon without an electronic brain. It's a sad fact!

I cannot go to the store without putting down my list in the phone as a reference when I get there. There is no way I will get everything I intended to get otherwise. Thank God for technology!

Even during the writing of this book, there were many times when I would lose my train of thought right in the middle of a thought. I think I cleaned them all up as I have gone along, but if you notice any, just have a chuckle over it and know where it came from. Chemo brain just really hampers your cognitive abilities in general. That can appear in any part of your life. As frustrating as it is, try to cut yourself a break and realize that it's chemo's fault, not yours.

8. RADIATION THERAPY

Radiation therapy is widely used in the treatment of breast cancer. While Chemo seeks out random cells floating around in the body, radiation therapy is much more targeted. It basically seeks to zap and bust up clusters of cancer cells. So it typically aims at tumor sites, lymph nodes or along mammosite which is the incision line for a mastectomy. It typically is done 5 days a week over a course of several weeks. It is significantly easier to tolerate than chemo, but it is not without its own unique challenges.

There are several portions of radiation prep. First, they will do tests to determine exactly where they want to aim the therapy. They may also prepare a mold for you to ensure that you are in the same position every treatment. That part of the process was actually fun! When they made mine, they basically poured this stuff that looks like pancake batter into a plastic pillow case. I laid on the table, and the stuff rose up around and conformed to my body. It was warm and comfy. I could have stayed there reclining all day if they let me. Unfortunately, it doesn't stay warm. When you go for treatment, the mold is usually freezing cold, along with the room itself, which is lovely considering you are likely to be half dressed in a hospital gown. I asked for lots of blankets to help stay somewhat comfortable.

I came up with two invention ideas from this process. One is to make custom beach chairs out of the pancake batter stuff (I am sure there is a more technical term for it). Think of reclining on the seashore with a gentle breeze blowing at the hair that you grew back in a chair that literally hugs you as you relax! Ahhhhh. The second is to find a way to keep that stuff warm during treatment. I am curious as to whether or not any of the readers of my book have the inventors bone in them. Feel free to throw me a cut when you make your millions, ok? Thanks!

An important note: if your radiation comes at time when you are wearing head coverings, (i.e. radiation following chemo), make sure you wear whichever head covering is most comfortable for treatment when you have your mold made. Alternatively, it would be perfectly fine to wear nothing on your head at all to treatment. My doctor wanted me to wear the same hat to every treatment because if I wore something different (a wig or a different hat), it could theoretically shift your angles in the mold, and change where the treatment is hitting you. Radiation requires precision in order to hit the appropriate places in your body. I never thought of that until they told me. I guess that's where their experience is helpful.

Also, as part of the prep is the radiation tattoos. I laughed and teased my mother that who would have every thought that she and I would have gotten matching tattoos one day! My father was none too pleased. Go figure… All joking aside, they really are not a big deal. They mark you so that they line you up the same way for each treatment. The tattoos only look like someone dotted your skin with a blue ball point pen. Most people will never notice you have them. Having them done basically feels like a quick needle stick which you probably are very used to at this point anyway, so no worries.

The most common and fairly obvious side effect is radiation burn. Exposure to the radiation is cumulative and over time, can create some pretty intense skin reactions. There are steps that can help mitigate the reaction. There are several creams that can be applied to help the skin heal. Your doctor can make recommendations on which would be best for your skin. Be aware though that the creams are thick and goopy. They will likely ruin your clothes. Head on over to walmart and buy a bunch of cheapie tank tops or t-shirts. Do not wear anything good to radiation because you will only end up having to toss it anyway. It's important to ask the doctor to show you exactly where they will be treating you ahead of time. I didn't do that and didn't realize they were treating lymph nodes along my collar bone until about 3 weeks into treatment when I got an intense burn/reaction. I had been only applying the cream to areas where I knew I was being treated: the boobs and underarms. Oops!

Depending on how severe your burns are, don't be surprised that it may take a while for them to heal and for the discoloration to go away. I had spots on my collar bone for at least 6 months after treatment. I remember someone asking me if it was a bruise, that it looked like someone tried to choke me. Nice, real nice! Eventually, it went from searing reddish purple, to a deep pink, to a tan color, and is almost unnoticeable now.

The other main side effect of radiation is fatigue. It's nowhere near the same caliber of fatigue that you face during chemo. I would describe it to be more of a weariness by the end of each day. Basically, your body is working overtime to repair the skin and healthy tissue during treatment, so it takes a toll on your energy level. I remember needing to go to bed earlier and just feeling wiped out during treatment. It's very manageable though. You will likely be able to go about your normal routine, just with a little less pep in your step. In my case, I went to work every day, and went to treatment during my lunch hour.

A side effect that might take you by surprise is that you might end up with some sore muscles in your arms and back during treatment. When you go for breast radiation, you will have to lay with your arms up over your head for the duration of the treatment. It's likely a position you are not used to, and so your arms might get tired and sore. Also, your back might get a little sore from lying still on a board every day for a few weeks. This obviously will subside as time goes on, and is nothing to be concerned about.

One other side effect that I encountered that was unexpected was radiation irritation of the throat. Because I was radiated along the collar bone (due to lymph node involvement), some radiation leached into my throat and caused issues. It was uncomfortable and made eating a bit unpleasant, but not seriously painful. It also caused my stomach to be aggravated. I learned that contrary to popular belief, radiation can occasionally cause low grade nausea. My medical oncologist laughed when I mentioned this to him. He said the radiation oncologists like to let the medical oncologists get the bad rep for causing you nausea, but truth be told, either treatment can make it happen. Although, much like the fatigue, it is nothing like what you will experience with chemo.

Also, here's something that you might not have thought about unless it happens to you or if someone tells you. Having gained weight during chemo, I was anxious to lose it as soon as possible once I started feeling better. I didn't discuss this with my doctor, I just started watching and exercising. I was so excited because I was doing great losing the weight. One day, about halfway through my treatment plan, the tech who I was working with quietly said to me, "have you noticed that you are, um, shrinking?" nodding to my pink radiated girls. Proud as can be, I said, "oh yes, you can tell? I have been dieting" Her eyes grew wide as saucers and said, "please talk to the doctor about it. He might not want you to continue." Shocked, I said ok, and then when I saw him after treatment that day, I asked him why. He said, when you are losing weight successfully, it can obviously change your size. That in turn messes up with the radiation plan because as I mentioned about the head covering, radiation is very based on angles. If your body shape changes, it can affect where the dose of radiation is going.

Dang! I had to chuckle because I have NEVER had a doc tell me to stop losing weight before. And I had good momentum going, so that stunk. I stopped my diet and have yet to really get myself back on track. GAH! Moral of the story? Tell your doctor if you are considering doing something like this. Don't just take it on yourself.

Another potential risk to be aware of is the risk of organ damage from radiation. Oh fun! My radiation oncologist warned me that the lungs can sustain injury from the treatment. As much as the doctors try to avoid it, there may not be the option if they radiate the chest wall. A certain amount of radiation may hit the lungs. Often times, the side effects from that manifest down the road. I developed a lovely case of asthma from my treatment. It didn't develop into a problem until a few months out of active treatment. Seriously, why is it that treatments fix one problem, but sometimes screw up something else? Sometimes, we just can't win for trying. It's highly annoying.

9. OTHER TREATMENT OPTIONS

The positive side of the commonplace nature of breast cancer being is that there is endless fundraising, countless studies and constant research about this disease. Treatment is evolving practically daily, with greater results. There are so many additional treatment options that have been discovered over the years that are supplemental to the standard surgery, chemo and radiation that can help improve the chances of a positive health outcome for so many women.

Much of the research has been focused on understanding the characteristics of breast cancer tumors. The more they know about tumors and how they proliferate, the more they can learn how to stop them from growing. At the time of this writing, there are 3 characteristics that they look for in the pathology of a tumor: Estrogen receptors, Progesterone receptors and the expression of the HER2/neu protein.

If any of these three characteristics exist, it would be referred to as hormone positive (for each estrogen and progesterone) and HER2 positive. The presence of these characteristics in your tumors add an extra layer of treatment that can help fight the disease. If none of these are present, that is what is called "triple negative" breast cancer. My cancer was ER and PR positive, Her2 negative. My mother was triple negative.

If the breast cancer is either estrogen receptor or progesterone receptor positive, that is considered hormone driven and can be treated several ways. Basically, the way I see it, for hormone positive breast cancer uses your hormones like little snack packs, and just keeps noshing away as it grows and grows. Given that, the doctor's goal often is to reduce the amount of food that the tumors are snacking on. Basically, these types of treatment put the cancer cells on an extreme diet with the intention of killing them via starvation. (This is not the technical description. This is just how I found it most easy to understand in my non-medically inclined head). There is a greater discussion around hormone positive cancer in the chapter

There is one primary known way to go after HER2 positive breast cancer: a very cool drug called herceptin. Basically, it intercepts the HER2 protein from binding to and feeding the cells. Think of it as a really good goalie in soccer. It blocks the protein from getting hooked up to cells and causing them to proliferate. The main down side is that herceptin can cause heart damage. (Seriously, why does everything have to have a frikking side effect? Ying and yang I suppose, but what a pain!) Doctors closely monitor the heart function of patients on herceptin to ensure they are safe.

I have to say, one thing that really fascinated me during the process was just how amazing science really is. I cannot tell you how many times during this process I thought to myself, "Who the hell figures this stuff out?" In this case, it was an awesome doctor named Dr. Dennis Slamon. He was an oncologist who studied breast cancer, discovered the Her2 protein and developed a way to block it. He's so cool, they made a Lifetime movie after him. That's when you know you are a big deal!

On the hormone side, there are several different approaches that can help. One of the most common is Tamoxifen which is inhibits estrogen from feeding cancer. It's particularly used in pre-menopausal women because the estrogen is still being generated by the ovaries. Depending on the levels of estrogen, there also is a couple of drugs that shut down ovarian function. This tends to have more severe side effects than Tamoxifen. The primary side effects of both are akin to menopause. Oh joy... Hot flashes, muscle cramps, insomnia, slowed metabolism (i.e. a huge pain in the butt for the purposes of losing weight.), mood swings, extra hair growth in weird places, higher risk of endometrial cancer, crazy stuff like that. I clearly remember when I told my husband Steve I would be taking it. He looked it up and replied facetiously "oh that sounds like a fun drug".

In post-menopausal women, doctors might opt for a class of drugs called aromatase-inhibitors. Essentially, when a woman is menopausal, her ovaries are not producing estrogen like they used to, which in the instance of hormone positive breast cancer is a good thing. That doesn't reduce all sources of estrogen though. Estrogen can manifest in other ways in the body through the development of aromatase, like through the adrenal glands. The drugs prevent the body from producing this form of the hormone, thereby further reducing the food supply for the cancer. It does seem that the side effects with the AIs are less than those for tamoxifen. Obviously, this all varies from one woman to another.

The lack of estrogen can do some not so fun things. Aside from the unpleasant but manageable side effects listed above, it can also contribute to heart issues and to bone loss. It's important to work with your medical team to monitor these issues. Adopting a healthy lifestyle can help mitigate it some.

One other extreme option to reducing estrogen is to have your ovaries removed. This obviously is not something to be taken lightly depending on your family status and desire to bear children in the future. A reason to consider it is that there is a link between breast cancer and ovarian cancer, especially if you have one of the BRCA gene mutations. One might want to remove them as a precautionary measure. Be mindful though, if you opt for this, it will throw you head first into surgical menopause, and there is no going back.

Additionally, they are finding that osteoporosis drugs are having a huge benefit here. They are not only helping with the bone loss, the medical community is starting to investigate if these drugs are boosting survival rates and reducing the risk of recurrence and metastasis. Pretty exciting! You have to love science and its ongoing development. It's amazing what research can uncover.

10. ALL IN THE FAMILY

Truth be told, a cancer diagnosis affects everyone in your world. The only thing that is as crappy as being diagnosed with cancer yourself is having someone you love being diagnosed. When I found out I had breast cancer, we had no family history. I was the first one, therefore, you can imagine our collective shock. I was 34 years old, so breast cancer was nowhere on my radar screen.

The interesting thing about history is that it is constantly being written. When an immediate family member is diagnosed with breast cancer, the odds of the other women in the family getting breast cancer doubles. With that said, right smack in the middle of my radiation treatment, my mom was diagnosed with breast cancer as well. Just great! Talk about adding insult to injury. The good news is, they caught her breast cancer at Stage I and we firmly believe this wouldn't have been caught until way later if I had not been diagnosed. There is something to be said for being watched like a hawk. In the course of less than a year, we went from no family history to a very strong one. Oddly enough, we are both BRCA negative.

The big mystery is how that happened. Considering the lack of the BRCA gene mutation in our DNA, it leaves other possible causes. Either there is another genetic link that they have not yet discovered, or perhaps ours was caused by environmental factors. We did spend a substantial amount of years living under the same roof, sharing the same water supply, food sources, etc. So who knows. I will leave that to the scientists to figure out. Regardless of why it happened, the fact is it happened, and we had to deal with it.

Needless to say, my first reaction was to ask "haven't we as a family gone through enough?" I got incredibly angry, way more angry than I did when I was diagnosed. It wasn't fair that mom now had to go through this after all she went through watching me. She experienced so much stress and heartache over my cancer. The toll treatments take on a family is tremendous, and needless to say, when it happens to several family members, it feels pretty catastrophic.

Now that we have both gone through treatment, it's definitely strange, but interesting for me to reflect on the fact that I have been on both sides of the fence. I hope it made me a bit more compassionate and supportive of her. Not that I wouldn't have done whatever she needed had I not gone through it, but I could truly relate to every experience she had, and that made it easier to support her emotionally because I understood her experiences in the way no one else ever could. As I have said previously, there is a comfort when you connect with someone who truly gets your experience. Being able to be that for my mom was a huge blessing for me. Perhaps this was the unique chance for me to slightly repay her for all of the love and guidance she gave me through the years.

While much of this book focuses on what it is like as a survivor, there is a whole concept of co-survivor that is worth discussing. It's very different to experience cancer as a co-survivor than as a survivor. Co-survivors are pretty much anyone significant in your support system. It could be spouses, boyfriends, girlfriends, children, parents, siblings, friends. It is anyone who is going on this journey with you. It's basically the people who love you and who cannot help but be directly impacted by your cancer and treatment.

Co-survivors (myself included now) often struggle with a wide mix of emotions. Often times, they feel frustrated and helpless because they can't stop what is happening to their loved ones, and they can't really fix it. Watching someone you love suffer through treatments is heart wrenching. There is no getting around that fact. However, there are can be some positive to be found if you look hard enough, and there certainly are things you can do to help your loved one.

Here are some thoughts for co-survivors that might help alleviate that helpless feeling. First off, it's important to let your cancer survivor know that you are there for them. This seems basic, but in their new world, everything feels uncertain and foreign. It's very disorienting. While it's true that they should know that you are there, hearing it is important. Don't be afraid to talk to them about cancer, but even more importantly, don't be afraid to talk to them about anything other than cancer. Truth be told, it gets really old talking about medical issues all day long. At some point, it becomes refreshing to talk about regular life, real-world issues, drama and triumphs. Real life can be a welcome distraction, trust me.

Cancer tries its best to consume the world, but the world keeps turning even though someone has the disease. For me, it was important to see life continued. It gave me a sense of relief when I saw that life outside my small corner didn't change much. So when friends called to vent about normal life problems, at first they expressed feeling weird about doing so, but truthfully, it felt good to me. I liked my life before cancer, so the best thing someone could do for me was to give me glimpses of that life again. I didn't want to be protected or treated as fragile now that I had this disease. I just wanted to feel like myself.

I vividly remember some co-survivors having happy experiences going on in their lives, and telling me that they felt strange having their joy juxtaposed to what I was experiencing. They almost wanted to hide it so as to seem not boastful. To me, I found this silly and I promptly told them so. I didn't want the world to be miserable just because I was going through something not so fun. In fact, their happiness gave me something positive to enjoy too. It was wonderful to have something hopeful and exciting to boost me up when much of what I was experiencing was sad and stressful.

Co-survivors often want nothing more than to take away the pain and soothe the fears, but often they don't know how. This can add to their angst. This is where communication is important. Don't be shy about expressing your needs as a patient, and don't feel badly about conceding that you will need help along the way. There is no shame in that. This is a very hard concept for many women to accept at first. It took time for me to learn how to speak up and let people know what my needs were. Letting them help you can be therapeutic for them.

Prior to cancer, I was the one who took care of many people in my life. I suspect most breast cancer patients and survivors take a similar role in their lives, after all, that's what wives, moms, sisters and friends do! While going through treatment, I often felt guilty for being limited in my abilities. This was particularly compounded being a mom. I have always been my son's primary caretaker. My husband is a wonderful daddy and is very involved with raising our son, but when it came down to it, Mommy is his main go-to person. When I was worn down by surgery and treatment, and couldn't do it broke my heart. However, I reminded myself that the purpose of being weak now was to be stronger later. If I pushed through my treatment, I would be able to have more quality time with my son and husband in the future. That was the main motivator and helped allay the guilt I felt on the days when I was physically unable to get out of bed. Given that I had to aggressively plow through treatment, I needed to rely on others to pitch in with my son to keep things as normal as possible for him with the exception of me being out of commission.

In the early days, I was so grateful for those who took it upon themselves to find ways to help, offering to hang out with my son or cook some meals. However, I found the majority of my support system was just as blindsided as I was, and didn't know how to support me. It was too overwhelming and scary for them to figure out what would help. I can understand that. They were taking on new roles too, and those roles were very undefined. In time, I learned to tell them what I needed. I had to learn to ask for help with things that were so basic: house work, driving me around at times when it wasn't safe for me to do so myself, cooking, caring for my son. Once they were able to understand my needs, it made things easier for me and for them. Co-survivors want so much to be able to contribute in some way.

As a co-survivor, it's important to think about the basics. As I explained, it may be hard for a cancer patient may not tell you what they need. They may not even know themselves what would be helpful. Here's what I can tell you, just do anything. Pitch in and do some chores, or consider getting them a gift certificate to a cleaning service. There actually is a non-profit organization out there called "cleaning for a reason" where local cleaning services will volunteer to provide their services to cancer patients. This could be a tremendous help because when going through treatment, the patient's energy will be terribly low at several points along the way. Cook a meal or send them frozen meals that can be quickly heated. Or do something simple like send a card or flowers. You have no idea how much a little gesture like that can brighten the day of someone going through treatment. When a woman is going through treatment, it's a very isolating feeling because the rest of the world is going about it's normal life, and we really can't participate. It was such a boost for me when people would randomly let me know they were thinking of me. I was grateful for every card that was sent to me. I kept every one and read them now and again when I need a pick me up.

I had a cousin come stay with me for a week after my surgery because she had gone through it with her mom. She knew what to expect and wasn't afraid to help. I am eternally grateful for her help and fantastic sense of humor at such a crazy time. Having her there was a huge comfort to me, and when it was time for her to go back home (she lives a 5 hour flight away), I was sad, but so very appreciative. The sacrifice she made for me was tremendous.

Some people helped with entertaining my son on the days that I knew I was going to be particularly weak. Some people simply provided awesome comic relief. Some played chauffeur for me on treatment days. One headed up a team of 75 to walk in my honor at an event for American Cancer Society, and baked the most amazing cake for us to celebrate. Some people just came and hung out with me when I was down, even if that meant just laying down watching mindless tv with me. Many people sent wonderful, thoughtful gifts which were such an awesome surprise and truly lifted my spirits. Some just treated me like I was normal, and that was such a comfort to me. Some people wore bracelets to show they were thinking of me. My one brother (who's organized professional wardrobe is legendary in some parts of the east coast) always work a pink shirt to work on treatment days. My two beautiful nieces made me homemade cards and donated their hair to locks of love to show their support. That really touched my heart and made me cry tears of pride. It's wonderful to see those beautiful girls learning to take a negative situation and do something good with it. They learned compassion young and it will only make their lives more amazing as they grow.

One thing to remember is that co-survivors might also benefit from counseling services. It is so traumatic and stressful to watch someone you love going through a journey like this. As much as it impacts the survivor, it also impacts the family and friends. The best thing a co-survivor can do is take care of themselves, and keep themselves strong and healthy so that they can be there to support their loved one. It's not a sign of weakness for a co-survivor to see help or resources. Co-survivors are suffering too and rightfully so.

11. YOUNG SURVIVORSHIP

Let's face it. Getting breast cancer just plain sucks at any age. Admittedly, though, there is an added stress associated with getting breast cancer young. There's a heightened feeling of unfairness. In my experience, the majority of women who are diagnosed young seem to fall into one of two categories: they either are BRCA positive or they have hormone positive tumors that were fed by pregnancy or post-partum changes. In my experience, there are two primary causal factors in early onset breast cancer: genetic mutation (BRCA 1 or 2) or hormones gone crazy.

During 2004-2008, the median age at the time of breast cancer diagnosis was 61 years[ii]. I was 34 when I received my diagnosis. I can't lie. That part really ticked me off! Feeling like I was in such a small minority of women who got brought into this club at an early age was so hard. Believe it or not though, young survivors are more common than you would think. In 2011, the American Cancer Society indicates there were approximately 13,100 new cases of breast cancer in women under the age of 40. While that is a small number compared to the 288,130 women of all ages, it's still more than most people realize[iii].

The problem is that except for high-risk women, there is really not much preventative screening available. In fact, there are some government entities that if they had their way would push back mandatory mammogram coverage to the age of 50! Talk about an outrage! Clearly, this group isn't in touch with the lives of those who are affected by this disease, and are ignorant to the fact that young women can get it. Or they consider us to be the "disposable" minority. As you might imagine, my head nearly exploded when I heard this!

With the lack of screenings, it's extremely important for women to do self-exams. We have to be proactive about our own health and not leave it up to some panel to dictate what the appropriate age to get breast cancer is. Routine mammograms are only covered by insurance if the patient is considered high risk due to family history or known genetic mutations. Because of this, unfortunately, women who are diagnosed young tend to be a higher stage because they don't often get the benefit of early detection. Many times, women in this age bracket find the cancer themselves. Generally, a Stage 0 or 1 tumor is not palpable, and therefore may not be picked up during self-exams. Imaging is what usually detects this disease when it's tiny.

We all know that breast cancer is increasingly more treatable the earlier that it is detected. Considering the lack of early detection tools available to most young women, that fact doesn't give us much comfort, as we don't have the tools available that older women do. We are more likely to find it later on our own. In our favor though, given our youth and likely reasonably good health status (aside from the big red cancer flag in our medical files), doctors can be more aggressive and may have more options for treating us as our bodies may be able to handle more and recover better than women of advanced age. They might be able to give us higher or more frequent doses of chemo or radiation. They might have more surgical options available. Youth does have its advantages, I suppose.

Anyone who gets a breast cancer diagnosis will likely encounter the "why is this happening to me" question at some point. Truth be told, I believe that emotion is more magnified when you are dealing with the fact that you aren't the "appropriate" age for your disease. Given that, there's an added feeling of unfairness that comes with getting diagnosed at practically half the age of when the statistics say you should. Especially when our own medical community says the chance of us getting it at that age is so slim that we aren't eligible for routine screenings. When it comes to being diagnosed with cancer, no one wants to be that rare person who defies the odds in a negative way. Talk about a crappy way to be exceptional!

Women in this age bracket may encounter different fears and decisions than the average breast cancer patient. Sometimes, there may be the added pressure to look a certain way when you are younger (although I am certain that body image issues can exist at any age). Some women may be struggling with how you get back into the dating game and eventually into an intimate relationship after breast cancer, especially if you opted for a mastectomy. If you are struggling with how you feel about your own body, it's certainly natural to feel that it may be difficult to find a partner who accepts your differences when you have that very struggle yourself. The fear is normal, but the truth is, there are wonderful people out there who will love you regardless of what you have been through. And if you are lucky, you will find someone who loves you BECAUSE of what you have been through. Yes, there are people out there like that! But remember, sometimes, it takes loving yourself, battle scars and all first. No relationship will fill your heart if you don't know how amazing you are.

Another potential concern that plays into young survivorship is fertility. The majority of women who get diagnosed with breast cancer are post-menopausal, so obviously, this isn't an concern for them. But for us young'uns, it can be a big deal. It is important to know that there are some courses of treatment that can have an effect on your future ability to conceive and carry a child. This can be especially tricky if your cancer happens to be hormone positive, like mine was.

While this might be the furthest thing from your mind in the midst of all of the oncological talk, it's important to consider. I highly recommend speaking to your doctors, and understanding the potential impact of the treatment protocol that you choose. Discuss not only the potential impact of treatment, but what options you have for preserving your fertility. There are a lot of options out there, but you will likely need to act quickly if you would like to exercise any of them. Many of them require decisions and actions before you get into chemo or hormonal therapy. I know this is the last thing you want to be thinking about while faced with a huge mountain to climb, but take the time to think through what you want to do. You have control over this part, take some peace of mind in making the best decision for you and your unique circumstances.

Treat these decisions as you would treat any others you make during this time, they are as important and as personal as all of the rest. Only you can determine what is best for you. No one can make that decision for you. Don't feel pressured into choices by anyone but yourself. This is about as personal as it gets. It affects your future and your body. Others may (and probably will) have opinions on this topic, but this is not a time to worry about those opinions. It's a time to listen to your heart and decide from there. It's certainly fine to understand the different options and to gather facts from different sources. I strongly encourage that because you will face some big decisions and ultimately you need to be comfortable with what you decide. Ultimately, this impacts you more than anyone else in this world, and only you can decide if you want to preserve your fertility or not. It's your body.

Related to the issue of fertility is the very real possibility of early onset menopause, especially if your cancer is hormone driven.

First off, you should know that chemo can cause your periods to stop temporarily (or sometimes permanently). Certain chemo drugs basically stop the ovaries from producing estrogen and often eggs while you are receiving them. It took me two chemo cycles to bring my girly cycles to a screeching halt. I can't lie, I was a little psyched about that. Adios tampons! There is a small blessing in all this craziness after all. No more cramps, not more PMS (although it does get replaced by menopause's own version of it, which is equally as fun).

Subsequent to the chemo induced menopause, you and your medical team might look at your case and decide that permanent menopause is the way to go. The reproductive system sometimes does come back into action when chemo concludes. However, sometimes, it might be prudent to prevent that from happening. Drugs like Tamoxifen and Lupron might be used to suppress the estrogen and ovaries. Think of it this way, in some cases, the estrogen is like fish food for tumor cells. So the less you have in your body, smaller the chances that cancer can grow.

Additionally, some women (myself included) opt to have the ovaries removed. There are two main reasons a woman might elect to do so. The first is that there is a link between some breast cancer and ovarian cancer. The second reason is, the ovaries are the largest producer of estrogen in the body, which as I just mentioned can be problematic if you are trying to starve any cancer floating around. This can be an extremely difficult choice if you are interested in preserving your fertility, and obviously can be emotional.

Menopause is about what you would expect. The hot flashes are annoying. Mine tend to be worse at night. I can feel them coming on too, which sometimes helps me to get a grip on them before I am a full flash mode. It feels like a weird tingly feeling on my face and skin and then Wham! Someone jacks up the high to blast. Ugh. I find that cool water or ice on my wrists and arms sometimes helps fend it off, but not all the time. In my case, it feels like someone cranked up a heat lamp and is blaring at my face until I start sweating. Just delightful. Ugh!

Night sweats and insomnia are common in menopause which is annoying. Lack of sleep is less than pleasant and unfortunately, has a carry-over affect into the next day. This can lead to crankiness, which of course is exacerbated by the fun that is menopause moodiness and emotional reactions. And let me tell you, this is the last thing you need when you are post-treatment. Many feelings are way more heightened, including fearful thoughts.

Other fun side effects of menopause are a slowed metabolism, which is a real pain when you want to lose weight. Then there is the need for extra tweezing. I won't get into detail here, but you can imagine the fun that comes with this category! There is also the slowing of your libido (or in some cases, bringing it to a screeching halt). I wonder if maybe this is God's way of making the men suffer through this with us. Some women also are more susceptible to muscle cramps such as Charlie horses. I am grateful for small miracles. This is one side effect I have yet to get.

One other concern for women in menopause is osteoporosis. This can be accelerated based on some of the meds you might be taking. But there is a pretty cool upside to this. As I mentioned earlier, recent findings are showing promising results in the use of osteoporosis drugs in breast cancer survivors. This extends beyond just fixing osteoporosis. It also appears that such meds might also have a preventative effect on the bones and seem to be linked to reduced risk of metastasis! Woohoo! Talk about exciting.

As with any other "change of life", menopause is linked to mood swings. Couple that with a cancer diagnosis, and really, I don't know how anyone could expect us to be sane, rational people! Hormones wildly swinging up and down (more likely down), emotions about having the big c. It's a wonder we all don't end up in padded rooms. But we are strong and we manage through. It's part of life, and we can't change that we got the diagnosis, we can only do our best to recognize how it might affect us emotionally and do our best to manage under the circumstances. My point is, do not be surprised if you are more emotional than usual. Your body is going through a roller coaster of epic proportions, one that would make even amusement park enthusiast wide-eyed and slightly sea-sick.

One of the extra crappy parts about this type of menopause is that the options that most women use to treat the symptoms are usually not recommended for those of us who have had hormone-driven cancers. Basically, the whole approach to managing the symptoms is to introduce synthetic hormones or consuming products that are designed to help boost hormones that naturally wane off during menopause. Of course, that's a bad idea when you want those hormone levels to stay low. So unfortunately, we are stuck here in menopause land for a while.

There is an upside though. All women go through menopause at some point. It's a fact of life. At some point, the side effects drop off once our bodies adjust. We get that crap over with sooner than the rest. Think of how fun it will be to laugh at your friends while they are fanning themselves, dripping in sweat in about 15 years! You will be comfy and cool as a cucumber, sipping a fruity drink, and they will be out of their minds and sweaty.

Paramount to fertility and other girly issues, there is also just the plain old fear of dying young. Let's not kid ourselves. Breast cancer is very treatable, but it can also be deadly. While the vast majority of women who get diagnosed with early-stage breast cancer do very well in treatment, and go on to live long, healthy, disease-free lives, that unfortunately does not apply to everyone. Susan G. Komen, whose name has become ubiquitous with the breast cancer was 33 when she was diagnosed and 36 when she lost her battle. She was one of us! This is a sobering reality. However, her sister, Nancy Brinker, who also diagnosed in her late 30s, survived long-term and went on to found Susan G Komen for the Cure. Ms. Brinker's amazing successes shows that women who get early onset breast cancer can in fact live impactful, awesome lives. She made it her life's work to eradicate the disease through research and education. So, here are two brave, beautiful young women cancer survivors, juxtaposed, impacting the world in their own intertwined way.

The fear is real. It's valid. We can only control so much with cancer. We can live the best lifestyle based on the recommendations of the medical community, and then the rest is left up to fate. That kind of sucks! But it's a reality. It's hard to accept that we don't crystal ball. This is where the serenity prayer comes in handy. We need to learn to do the best with what we can control, and somehow learn to peacefully accept the rest. Trust me, this is no small feat. I cannot say it is something I have mastered. It is something I work on nearly every day of my life.

Many women who are diagnosed with breast cancer young may be mothers. That certainly adds to the list of challenges we face. I fell into this category. My son was two and a half when I was diagnosed. While I laid there on the table being biopsied, he and my husband were my first thought. How would they manage? I wasn't so much worried about me and what I would endure. I was worried about them. How would this affect them? Would it cause them sadness or fear? It broke my heart to think that I would be the cause of that. Would they be ok while I focused on my health?

Children can struggle seeing their mommies sick, and depending on their age, they may not understand what is happening. In my son's case, because he was so young, we didn't delve into the overall theme of cancer with him. We dealt with it symptomatically. We found that dealing with it that way was an age-appropriate approach. "Mommy's tired today" or "Mommy has boo-boos and can't pick you up" (yes, of course this broke my heart!). My favorite was "Mommy decided she wants to have a haircut like Daddy". Never was I more grateful to have a husband with a shaved head! My son was good with that and never once flinched at my baldness. In fact, he hated it when I wore the wig and often times asked me to take my hat off. Bless his little unaffected heart!

If you have children, it's up to you as to how you want to approach it with them. I think honesty within your family is a good thing, with perhaps some restrictions depending on the age you are dealing with. Cancer affects the whole family. Unfortunately, there is no getting around that. Treatment can take a while so it's not likely going to be something you can hide from your kids. Depending on their age and if you feel it's appropriate, you might want to considering getting them professional help managing their emotions. While this might sound crazy, you might also find that although it's a traumatic experience for all involved, it might really cultivate a compassionate side in your child. I noticed more and more that my son was in tune to people not feeling well or being sad. Once he picked up on that, he instinctually tried to make me smile or comfort me in his own way. Kids are so amazingly resilient. I think sometimes they handle a catastrophic situation better than we adults do. My son certainly did.

On a more practical front, younger women may have less medical coverage or life insurance than older women. We tend to think we are more invincible and tend to be less practical. I can tell you one of my biggest regrets was letting my life insurance lapse and not re-upping it when I had the chance. The December before I got diagnosed, I had intended on signing up for the supplemental life insurance policy during our open enrollment at work. It cost $100 for the blood work necessary to qualify for coverage. Considering it was Christmas time, money was a little tight, and I thought to myself, "No big deal, I'll just sign up next year." What a big mistake! By the time next year rolled around, no life insurance company wanted to touch me with a ten foot pole. I was now black listed as a cancer survivor and it will likely be another 5 or 10 years before anyone even thinks about granting me a policy. I was certainly penny-wise, pound-foolish. Please learn from me if it is possible!

12. LIFE AFTER ACTIVE TREATMENT

What you go through after a cancer diagnosis is traumatic. It's a big deal. No, wait. A huge deal! Don't belittle it and think that it's not. It affects you to your core. There is nothing you can do to prevent it from doing so. For me, I felt very betrayed by my body. It unnerved me that I had this demon growing inside of my breasts, and it was marching in a very dangerous direction, and I had no clue. This was a terrifying reality for me. That's the worst kind of enemy: an underhanded one! I personally think that cancer should be brought up on some kind of terrorist charges and banished for good! I thought I knew my body well, and I thought I was healthy. When I realized both of those assumptions were flawed, it really knocked me for a loop. That is very hard to recover from emotionally, or at least for me it was. And based on most of the survivors I have talked to, the emotional healing process takes a lot longer than the physical recovery.

Many women feel like they are unwillingly pushed out of the nest post treatment. That can be a daunting experience as well. There is a certain comfort that comes with seeing your doctor constantly. There's a safe feeling knowing that if anything weird pops up, you can pretty much address it immediately. It's a little scary to suddenly go months without seeing him or her. You will likely become close to your medical team. Over the course of treatment, you spend a lot of time with them. You will see them on a very regular basis, and it starts to become normal for you. Then when treatment ends, you stop cold turkey! Like anything else, this can produce anxiety. Sure, you will still have regular appointments with your doctor, but not nearly as regularly as you did during treatment. The time in between makes you feel a little lost, uncertain of yourself.

It takes a lot of work, time and patience to heal physically from a breast cancer battle. In reality, a breast cancer survivor is often very similar to a veteran returning from war. You still have glimpses of the person you were before you entered, but on the flip side, you are impacted, often traumatized by what you have experienced. Putting your life back together can be hard. Re-entering your life may make you feel tenuous. It's not uncommon to experience post-traumatic stress. Not unlike a Vietnam vet who fears land mines to this day, a cancer survivor may live in fear of recurrence or worse, metastasis. And certain things can trigger that fear to come back with a vengeance.

It's also a strange feeling when the rest of the world thinks that just because you are done with treatment that you are done with cancer. I remember people saying "yay! You're cured!" Well, thanks for your vote of confidence, but sadly, it's not so! Cancer recurrence and metastasis risk doesn't just vaporize the moment they remove the needle for your last infusion or you rub cream on your last radiation burn. As much as I would love to believe that and embrace it, I know it's not that easy. Even most oncologists agree that the use of the word "cure" with cancer is misleading at best, at least in the first few years following treatment. Every patient's journey unfolds over time, and none of us know where we will land.

Life doesn't go right back to normal once it's all over. It's hard to find where you fit in your new world. Things are different, no matter how much you want them to go exactly back to where they were before cancer. It can be a very strange feeling when you have an army rallied around you when you are in treatment, and suddenly once treatment ends, they go back to normal life, innocently assuming you are "all good" now. They often don't realize that once you take that last treatment, it's not over for you. Certainly, it's absolutely wonderful to have the rigors of treatment behind you, but much of the trauma remains. They mean well, but often, they don't realize any struggles that follow you beyond treatment. So you are left, feeling somewhat alone, to work through some of the more frightening emotions. I know many women who emotionally made it through treatment great, who only emotionally felt the effects months or even years later. Sometimes, your mind goes into self-preservation mode during treatment, but once you are out, your guard goes down, and the emotional trauma hits you like a ton of bricks.

After I finished treatment and was going to get my first set of scans, I outright refused to let my doctor do them until after a planned vacation. My family and I had been through enough and I knew that no one could completely guarantee me good news. Unless there was a guarantee, I didn't care how slim the chance was of there being a problem with the scans, I was not doing it. I was too afraid that there was going to be problem. The doctor obliged and scheduled them for the week I returned. Granted, it only ended up delaying those scans for a few weeks, so I am not suggesting pushing any tests out months.

Anytime there was a test coming up, I internally panicked. It was odd, there was part of me that wanted nothing more than to hear the words "no evidence of disease" but the route to get there always paralyzed me. Blood work, scans, it didn't matter: anything that could show any form of red flag terrified me. I remember being on the phone with my oncologist's office awaiting blood work for the first time. She paused while she pulled up my tumor marker report, my heart practically stopped.

The results were normal, but not before a wave of paralyzing terror washed over me.

For me, planning the future became incredible difficult. This was something I didn't expect. I previously was always thinking ahead about what was next in life. I was ambitious, and thought a lot about what my next career step would be, or how my family would continue to grow. I happened to be at a cross-road when cancer struck. My husband and I were planning to start trying for our second child. I had just made the decision that I wanted to stay with my current employer long-term and grow with them (which I am very grateful for because I learned I was quite blessed to work for a compassionate employer, something I never thought I would need). We were working with an architect to plan the expansion of our home. Then my life suddenly and violently jumped the tracks. In one fell swoop, my trust in my ability to plan anything was shattered.

After that experience, I had a planning phobia! I had a hard time thinking past my next appointment or test. I would constantly find myself saying things like "if my health holds out" when making plans. I became paranoid. Every ache and pain scared me. I remember someone telling me early on "oh, you have cancer? You know you will never get a head ache again, right?" At first I didn't understand what that meant. Then I realized, every ache and pain is not just your standard ache and pain anymore. Our minds want to go to the scariest place once we have been traumatized. If I had a cough, I would worry about metastasis to the lung. If I had a back ache, I was worried that it moved into my spine. Fear that followed me everywhere indeed! It's a crappy emotional side effect of this disease. It was something (and is still something) that I work have to work on emotionally to stay sane.

I remember having a conversation with my boss about my professional development. He was encouraging me and wanted to talk about what I could do to further my career and grow within the company. Most women (including myself a year prior) would have jumped at the opportunity to have such a discussion. I admitted to him that I was nervous to talk about my future with the company because what if something happened and I couldn't do those things we planned for me to do. At some point, I had to learn to let that fear go a bit and not limit myself and my future potential on the premise of "what if". But admittedly, that was hard. I didn't want to commit to something if there was a chance that I couldn't deliver. However, I had to try. I owed myself that much! Cancer didn't deserve the power to keep me stuck in fear. I worked too hard to get where I was in my life to let something like some stupid little cells having a party in my body stop me. It's funny, why is it the little things that scare us the most? In my case, bees, spiders, and cancer cells are way up there on the scary list. Go figure.

It's important to realize that your body also still may have recovering to do. Aside from the long term emotional side effects, of course there are also physical ones as well. It may be a while before your energy returns to its previous levels. Some women find that their digestive tract takes a while to bounce back.

You may have to adjust to a new physical appearance. In my case, smaller, perkier boobs! Woohoo! The ability to go braless was something that was never an option for me before. I always had to choose bra-friendly attire or deal with the discomfort of a strapless bra, which when you are a DD really is no fun. Strapless bras are no match for gravity.

Another change that I didn't expect: no nipples. Kind of weird, but not terrible. It's odd to look in the mirror and look like a life-sized Barbie doll. The upside is, I never have to worry about "high beams" when it's cold again. I cannot tell you what a relief that is. No more having to cross my arms as I walk around the office! Yes, see, there is always a silver lining!

It was super exciting when my hair grew back. And let me just say "chemo curl" is no joke! We are talking little orphan annie curls. My hair was long and straight before cancer. Now it's a giant ball of curls. People are kind and give me lots of compliments. It's very weird to have to learn a different way to style my hair when I did it a different way for 34 years. I haven't gotten used to it, but I am grateful to have hair, so I will take it with a smile.

One other bizarre long-term side effect that will follow you out of treatment is sun sensitivity. Your doctor will likely tell you that you need to be really careful in the sun after treatment for at least 2 years (Granted, we all should always be careful, but truth be told, we should do a lot of things and regardless of our best intentions, it does not always happen.) My radiation oncologist warned me that my skin would be way more sensitive to the skin following my treatment. I took this to mean I would burn more easily. I assumed it would be unpleasant, but not a huge deal. Boy, was I ever wrong!

About six months after completing radiation therapy, I found myself getting lax. I went out one Sunday afternoon in July and had forgotten the sunblock. I realized it when I got to my destination, and foolishly shrugged it off. I did not get sunburned that day. Instead, over the course of the next week, I learned the definition of photosensitivity and solar urticaria. Yes, it's about as fun as it sounds. Over the next few days, any skin that was exposed to the sun had a severe allergic reaction. Oh dear Lord! Itchy irritated hives everywhere that had been exposed to the sun! Talk about uncomfortable. Let me tell you, sunburn stinks, but it is NOTHING compared to an allergic reaction to the sun! Sadly, that was a lesson hard learned.

So, please, learn from my mistake! Cover up. Use sunblock. Don't find out the hard way like I did. I also recommend rash guard-style bathing suits for the summer. There are a lot of cute ones out there. Channel your inner surfer chick and get a few of these for your fun in the sun.

I also don't suggest ever going to a doctor's appointment alone again. First off, trust me when I tell you that your own thoughts are not the world's best company to a cancer survivor. Secondly, realistically speaking, the trauma of cancer, the potential for reoccurrence still exists, even beyond treatment. In all likelihood, you will be just fine, but you never know. I'm not looking to be the voice of doom, but rather the voice of practicality.

It's scary, and let's face it, there is always the possibility that you will hear something you don't like at an appointment. The first time I tried to go to my oncologists alone because I thought it was no big deal, I expressed concern for a lump I felt under my arm. He sent me right into ultrasound later that day. While they were setting the appointment up, I heard them on the phone with the insurance company getting approval. I heard the words, "and we would like to biopsy if necessary". My heart stopped, and it felt like the world crashed in on me, and my husband and parents were all an hour and a half away. So there I was, terrified and alone, in the middle of a full-blown panic attack. My sanity was hanging by a piece of dental floss, and I was by myself. Never again!

Think of it this way, at every appointment, they are going to discuss your health status. They are either going to say something that is going to put your mind at ease, or they are going to say something that is going to terrify you. If it's not good news, you are going to need someone to lean on. Better yet, if it is good news, then it would be wonderful to have someone with you to share it and celebrate with!

I worked for a long time (and continue to work with) a mental health professional who specializes in oncology to keep things focused and prevent my mind from going to that dark, frightening place. But it is not easy! There were some tricks that helped me. First off, like I said earlier, getting professional help is key. There are some wonderful people out there who specialize in working with cancer survivors. They have been trained in this. Let them do their job! I work with her to practice "mindfulness" as she calls it which is being aware of what I know to be true at any given moment. It's about being self-aware of my thoughts and really reigning them in before they get out of hand. Rather than speculate ahead to what my next test might show, I try to focus on what the most recent test showed.

Also, I try focusing on all of the things that I have done to treat this disease. I made decisions that I thought were best for my health and long term prognosis so I could feel like I have done all that I can do to fight this disease. I also have learned to stay of web browsers, and stick to only a very limited list of reputable sources for breast cancer information. There are too many horror stories out there, and it's easy to get swept away in them. The best thing to do is to focus just on the facts and to only get information from positive, professional sources.

I also continued to go to support groups after my treatment. It's interesting because a lot of the women in the groups can relate to that feeling of what happens to you after treatment. Several women I knew only went after they found themselves struggling post-treatment. The great thing about support groups is it's amazing how good it can feel to know you are not the alone in your issues. It's very validating to see someone nod knowingly when you talk about something you are experiencing, or even better, to hear someone else describe their challenges, and realizing they could be talking about your very story. I remember talking about some of the side effects I was having at my very first group that I thought were odd. I was so very relieved when I realized several other women had experienced the same thing. It was a comfort to be in a place where I was normal. Many people who have not actually experienced cancer for themselves really cannot relate, no matter how compassionate and understanding they are. It's an alternate universe that only those who live in it can really comprehend.

In time, the anxiety does ease. As you gain more time between appointments, your life becomes less about cancer. That is a truly wonderful feeling. It's amazing how even though we do gradually move away from the emotions of cancer, they can quickly resurface. A visit to the hospital, the smell of a soap you used during treatment or the sound of a significant song can trigger the memory and emotions in a heartbeat. While writing this book, I often revisited some of my notes and blogs that I wrote while I was going through treatment. Several times, I felt tears suddenly spring to my eyes while I read those passages. I was surprised and how quickly my heart went back and experienced those emotions all over again, even a year past treatment. I guess in some respects, you never really leave it behind. It's part of who we are as survivors. Those memories can't be erased. Sadly, this is one time when chemo brain would come in handy, but alas, it's not strong enough to overpower those memories. Unfortunately, they can't use some fun mind-erasing trick to help us eliminate the painful memories. All we can do is make an effort to focus on the present and the future.

In recent years, there has been a growing survivorship movement. In the information age, people have more data and research at their fingertips to make informed choices about their health. Survivors have become more proactive in their approaches post-treatment. Many (myself included) use the opportunity to change their lifestyle. While we cannot really control whether or not cancer will return, there are some things we can do to increase our overall chances of survival, not only from cancer, but from any disease.

There are no guarantees, as we ultimately learn, but there are things we can do to up our chances. To me, if there was any component of prevention that I could control, I had to take it. I needed it for peace of mind. One easy component is exercise. In April of 2012, the American Cancer Society issued new recommendations on exercise. They found that 150 minutes per week significantly reduced the risk of recurrence and death from breast cancer.[iv] To me, that number sounded scary, until I realized that it amounted to a half hour 5 times a week. That's really not so bad at all! To me, knowing that I was doing something to up my chances, something to fight back really empowered me (and motivated me to get my butt out of bed and hit the gym on the days when I really didn't feel like it).

Ask your medical team about working on a survivorship plan. Many can give you guidance on all that you can do to live healthier. This may include dietary changes in addition to exercise. Each survivor would have different needs, so it's important to work on a plan that is specific to you and your lifestyle. Some doctors can give you referrals to nutritionists and other specialists who can help you set your lifestyle path forward.

The important thing to remember is that none of us know the future. Whether we are cancer survivors, co-survivors, or just regular people who have not been affected by breast cancer, none of us have a crystal ball. We don't know what the next chapter in our lives will be. We do not know if we will ever dance with cancer again. What we can do is live our best lives. We can focus our energies on appreciating what we have today. Enjoy every minute of our lives because we are here, and we can! Just because we have experienced cancer, does not mean we cannot still experience good. That is when cancer wins... We win when we live our best life despite of cancer and laugh in its face.

Be well...

ABOUT THE AUTHOR

Nicole Briamonte Malato grew up in North Jersey, and now resides in Toms River, NJ with her husband and son. She is the proud daughter of two real life heroes – a retired Jersey City fire captain and a breast cancer survivor.

She had forgotten how much she enjoyed writing until she was diagnosed. It reawakened her inner storyteller, and hopes that her experience will help other women who are going through early stage breast cancer by sharing her authentic experiences, emotions and tips she learned along the way.

Her day job is a Human Resources Manager. Her writing was predominantly a side effect of chemo steroids, insomnia and a desire to make other survivors' lives a little more bearable and less lonely.

Endnotes

[i]

http://www.cancer.org/Cancer/BreastCancer/DetailedGuide/breast-cancer-risk-factors

[ii] Howlader N, Noone AM, Krapcho M, et al., eds. SEER Cancer Statis-tics Review, 1975-2008. Bethesda, MD: National Cancer Institute; 2011. http://seer.cancer.gov/csr/1975_2008/, based on November 2010 SEER data submission, posted to the SEER web site.

[iii]

http://www.cancer.org/acs/groups/content/@epidemiologysurve illance/documents/document/acspc-030975.pdf

[iv]

http://www.cancer.org/cancer/news/expertvoices/post/2012/04/2 6/new-healthy-living-guidelines-for-cancer-survivors.aspx

14968938R00068

Made in the USA
Charleston, SC
10 October 2012